To: Sharon ~

Thank you for
all your support!

☺ Tamara

Fertility Walk

*A Fertility Nurse's
Guide Along
Your Journey*

Tamara Tobias
Women's Health Care Nurse Practitioner

Fertility Walk

Tamara Tobias

www.fertilitywalk.com

Shine PR Etc.
www.shinepretc.com

Printed in the United States of America

First Edition: September 2015

Library of Congress Cataloging-in-Publication Data

(Print) 978-1-68222-321-5 (E-book) 978-1-68222-322-2

Dedication

This book is dedicated to my husband who never stopped believing.
To my incredible family for their support through the years and those
difficult times when they didn't know what to say. To my twin boys who
keep me on my toes and to my beautiful adopted daughter who makes
me laugh with her delight in everyday moments.

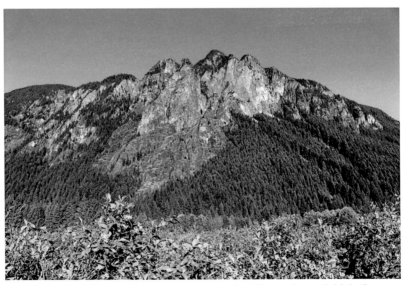

You CAN reach the top of a mountain. This is beautiful Mt Si
in my home of North Bend, Washington.

Special Thanks

I especially want to say "thank you" to the incredible patients I have met through my many years working in reproductive medicine. The stories they have shared with me, their triumphs, and their heartbreaks. We have laughed and we have cried together. Their strength, love, and determination continue to inspire me every single day.

To my son, Ryan, who wanted to contribute to this book. He has such passion for the outdoors, nature, and photography. He has captured striking pictures of the incredible beauty in the Pacific Northwest; many of these scenes are right from our own neighborhood.

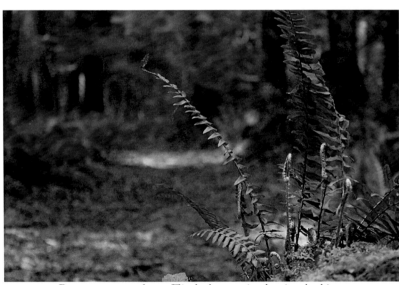

Beauty surrounds us. Find pleasure in the simple things.

Contents

About the Author

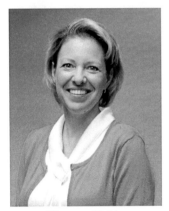

Tamara Tobias

Certified Women's Health Care Nurse Practitioner, Tamara Tobias has been offering care in reproductive medicine since 1997. Tamara obtained her Nursing degree from the College of St. Benedict in St. Joseph, Minnesota, Nurse Practitioner training at Harbor-UCLA, and Masters of Science Degree in Nursing from California State University, Long Beach.

Tamara is an active leader in the fertility community. She founded the Reproductive Nursing Association (RNA) of San Diego and Southern Orange County when she was working at the San Diego Fertility Center and was founding member of Seattle Tacoma Area Reproductive Society (STARS) when she moved to Seattle and began working at Seattle Reproductive Medicine (SRM). Both societies are non-profit organizations established to provide continuing education and networking for fertility experts.

Tamara is truly passionate about reproductive medicine both on a professional and personal level. On a professional level, some of her other accomplishments include:

- In 2007, she was elected on the Executive Council of the Society for Assisted Reproductive Technologies (SART)
- Active American Society of Reproductive Medicine (ASRM) member, serving on the SART Validation Committee and Chair of the Advanced Practice Provider Committee
- Past Chair of the Nurses' Professional Group (NPG) within ASRM
- Invited speaker at ASRM Annual Meetings and other professional conferences
- Published several articles in nursing newsletters and journals
- Recognized in 2014 as one of *Seattle Magazine's* Top Nurse Practitioners

On a personal level, Tamara's love for reproductive medicine stems from her own experience. After eight years of infertility and that emotional monthly turmoil, she and her husband conceived through IVF treatment. Those were very difficult times in her life and marriage, but her fertility journey did not stop there. Nine years later, she and her husband, Tim, adopted a beautiful little girl.

Life is so unpredictable with bends and roadblocks that seem impassable but Tamara's motto to this day is, "Believe in Miracles." In fact, this reminder is on a pin that she wears on her lab coat every single day.

Introduction

I understand all too well how difficult and painful the fertility journey can be. I also appreciate how overwhelming the barrage of medical information, terms, and ultrasounds can be. Although your intended path to parenthood may not be what you envisioned, you CAN achieve the family or resolution you desire.

The purpose of this book is twofold. I would like to help you gain a sense of control by better understanding your ultrasounds, menstrual cycle, treatment options, and procedures. We will discuss abnormal findings such as a cyst or fibroid and then all those questions that arise when a cycle IS successful. The back of this book has a list of common abbreviations used in reproductive medicine, included because all of the acronyms we use every day may be new to you. I hope to guide you through the process with easy-to-comprehend explanations and pictures. I am a visual person, and I know pictures really enhance my own learning.

My other intention is to walk with you along your journey because you are not alone. I can imagine all of the questions and worries that may be going through your mind, and I want you to think of me as a friend. I truly can relate to all of those mixed emotions, the good days and the bad days, and the days when you feel like just giving up. I remember asking myself, "why me?" After personal experience and working with so many women and couples who have struggled with infertility, just like you, and I am here to tell you there is hope.

The journey of infertility can be depicted in a variety of metaphors. It can be likened to a winter storm (wild, unexpected, frightening), a funeral (death of hopes and dreams), even a never-ending roller coaster (breathtaking and out of control). Maybe you can relate to these descriptions written by others on the infertility journey:

> Infertility feels like you are broken
> Infertility feels like a constant reminder that life is not fair
> Infertility feels lonely
> Infertility feels out of control'

My goal is to help you envision the journey of infertility as a walk. And although the definition of "walk" implies regularity and consistency, the walk we will take together will include many types of walking:

> **Plod**: walk slowly and heavily, as if reluctant or weary
> **Prance**: walk joyfully, as if dancing or skipping
> **Stumble**: walk clumsily or unsteadily, or trip
> **Tiptoe**: walk carefully on the toes or on the balls of the foot, as if in stealth

Truthfully, the trail we follow through infertility is not an easy one. We will stumble and fall, meander at times, and occasionally skip with joy. The key is that you will not be alone and you won't be without your walking tools; the following chapters are meant to serve as your compass, map, and mile markers. And me? Well, I'm your walking partner. As we take this walk together, **my ultimate intention for you is to find HOPE . . .**

> **Hope to alleviate fears and uncertainties**
> **Hope that you move forward on your journey**
> **Hope that your dreams will come true**
> **Hope that you will find peace within yourself**
> *Let's go take a walk . . .*

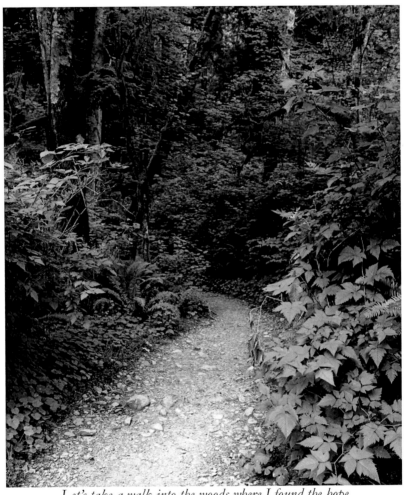

Let's take a walk into the woods where I found the hope
to get me through my journey.

Fertility Walk

A Fertility Nurse's Guide Along Your Journey

Chapter 1

What to Expect at Your Fertility Consultation

Take the first step . . .

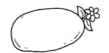

What to Expect at Your Fertility Consultation

Break Trail: (**verb**) – In winter, to hike in the lead position, forcing one's way through untrammeled snow. It is far easier to walk in the tracks of someone else who has already "broken" the trail.[i]

The infertility walk is not a new one; many have blazed the path before you and broken the trail. Whether you are freezing your eggs for fertility preservation or you have been trying to get pregnant for the last several months, or even years, you have taken a step in their tracks by reading this book or by making your initial appointment. Studies have shown that many people struggle with reproductive issues, but so many never reach out to make that first appointment or may never talk about it with others. Being able to conceive is supposed to come "naturally," and it is heartbreaking when attempts at pregnancy are unsuccessful or when our biological clock cannot wait.

The fertility journey is not easy, especially when the path isn't clearly marked. The stress of disappointment, worry, and confusion can render us immobile if we let them. Studies have looked at why people discontinue treatment when they have a good chance of pregnancy or even when fertility treatments are covered by insurance. They have found that people often give up along their journey because of the intense psychological or emotional burden. I strongly encourage you *NOT* to give up and talk to someone whether it is your provider, nurse, or coordinator about your concerns. Although your intended path to parenthood may not be what you had envisioned, you *CAN* achieve the family or resolution you desire.

Initial consultation

Your initial visit will most likely include a consultation with your provider to review your medical history, prior evaluation, and treatments you may have already done. A review of your partner's history (if applicable) will also be assessed.

This initial appointment may take 1-2 hours, so allow enough time in your schedule so you are not rushed. Additionally, some offices may perform a vaginal ultrasound and blood tests at your first visit even if you have recently done these tests with your OB/GYN provider.

A transvaginal ultrasound means that the ultrasound is performed with a probe inserted vaginally. This procedure does not hurt but may be a little uncomfortable. It is a quick procedure and emptying your bladder before the ultrasound often allows for better visualization. Please inform your provider if you have a latex allergy since latex probe covers are often used.

During the ultrasound, your fertility provider will focus on your antral follicle count, assessment of any ovarian cysts or uterine fibroids, and will get a general overview of your pelvic anatomy.

TRAILHEAD TIP:

Many providers perform a transvaginal ultrasound at your first appointment even if you already had one done by your OB/GYN provider.

After your initial consultation

Make sure to get your primary nurse or coordinator's name and phone number before you leave; you might think of more questions later. Some centers may also provide appropriate email addresses or a patient portal for follow-up questions. The first appointment may be a little overwhelming, and often there is a lot of information covered in a short period of time. I strongly encourage you to take the initiative and call or email your primary nurse or coordinator within 1-2 weeks after your initial consult. Your provider's plan will be outlined in your medical record, and your nurse or care coordinator can take you through the steps, especially if you are unsure of what to do next. Do not hesitate to reach out to your nurse or coordinator. They are there for you and building that relationship will only enhance your own experience.

Additionally, you will want to make an appointment with an OB/GYN for a routine annual exam. Make sure to give your fertility clinic the name and contact information for your OB/GYN. Often, your fertility doctor or provider will want to send them an update. If you do not have an OB/GYN provider, now is the time to get one.

Ask your fertility provider, nurse, or coordinator for referrals and get established with an OB/GYN provider before you are pregnant. Once you are pregnant, it will be much easier to make an appointment with an OB/GYN provider if you are already an established patient.

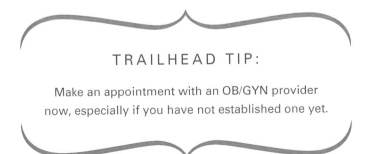

TRAILHEAD TIP:

Make an appointment with an OB/GYN provider
now, especially if you have not established one yet.

Follow-up

Your provider may order additional tests or procedures to be completed after your initial consultation or on certain days of your menstrual cycle. It is important for you to have a follow-up consultation with your provider to review the results. Your nurse or coordinator may or may not be able to give you the results and most centers prefer to review all of the findings with you in person and then discuss your individualized treatment plan.

Also, it is always important to have picture identification with you. Since fertility practices are dealing with gametes (eggs and sperm), patient identification is critical in this field of medicine.

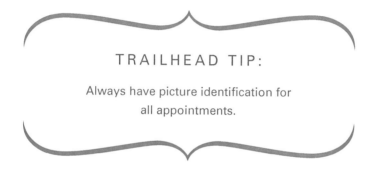

TRAILHEAD TIP:

Always have picture identification for all appointments.

The Fertility Evaluation

The 3 main components of a fertility evaluation are described below.

1. Ovulation and ovarian reserve

The menstrual cycle consists of a pre-ovulation (follicular) phase and post-ovulation (luteal) phase. Chapter 3 will review the menstrual cycle in more detail with accompanying ultrasound images to explain the different phases. Follicular refers to when a follicle (fluid surrounding the egg) is growing and getting ready to ovulate.

Ovulation can often be predicted with ovulation predictor kits (OPKs), which detect the luteinizing hormone (LH) surge prior to ovulation. Since progesterone increases after ovulation, a progesterone blood test one week after a presumed ovulation can also be used to confirm if ovulation indeed occurred.

If you get your period on a regular pattern every month, then you are likely ovulating. However, if your cycles are longer, like every 35-40 days, then you may have times when you are not ovulating. Oral ovulation medications can be used to overcome this irregularity. It is also important to let your provider know if you experience any abnormalities such as spotting in-between your periods or significant discomfort during your period or with intercourse.

Ovarian reserve refers to your egg supply and helps us predict how you may respond to fertility medications. I think it is fascinating that as women we are born with all of the eggs we will ever have yet, unfortunately, we cannot make more eggs. Tests to check your egg supply or ovarian reserve may include:

- Cycle day 3 FSH (Follicle Stimulating Hormone) and estradiol level
- Antimullerian Hormone level (AMH)
- Antral Follicle Count (AFC) ultrasound

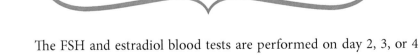

TRAILHEAD TIP:

Even if you have been on birth control pills for years and not ovulating, your egg supply is not being stored up. The normal process of ovarian aging is occuring and eggs still undergo cell death.

The FSH and estradiol blood tests are performed on day 2, 3, or 4 of your menstrual cycle. This blood test is done on the first days of your period because that is when your ovaries are normally quiet (not growing an egg), and your estrogen is low. FSH from your pituitary will then stimulate a follicle (egg) to grow. As we get older, the eggs become more difficult to stimulate, which results in a rise of FSH. An elevated FSH level is an indicator of decreasing egg supply or ovarian reserve and high FSH levels are used in the diagnosis of menopause. Estradiol is important as well because if the estradiol level is elevated, it can cause the FSH level to look incorrectly low. Therefore, you really need both a FSH and estradiol level to assess ovarian reserve. Sometimes the estradiol level may be high because a follicle is already starting to grow. The increased FSH level stimulates earlier onset of follicular growth and can result in short menstrual cycles; another indicator of diminished ovarian reserve.

Antimullerian hormone (AMH) is a hormone produced by cells that are in the small growing follicles, even the microscopic ones that we cannot see on ultrasound. This level decreases with age as the egg supply continues to deplete. This blood test may be done any time during your menstrual cycle and even if you are on birth control pills. However, long term use of birth control pills could suppress the AMH level and your provider may recommend discontinuation of them for 1 month and then repeat your AMH level if your first level was abnormally low.

The antral follicle count (AFC) is determined with a transvaginal ultrasound, which can be performed anytime during the menstrual cycle. The antral follicles are the small follicles seen on ultrasound, which I call "little wannabes." These antral follicles can be counted and the total number reflects your egg supply. See my illustration below. The average AFC is between 10-25 follicles total (both ovaries, not each one).

Age also plays a significant role with regards to fertility. As a woman gets older, her egg supply diminishes, and there are no medications that can increase egg supply. A mature egg must also divide its chromosomes in half in order to be fertilized. As we age, that process of dividing does not work as well and may result in chromosomal abnormalities. This explains why the miscarriage rate and risks of Down syndrome go up as we get older.

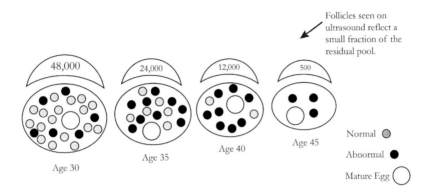

*Note, this illustration is an average. The quality of eggs diminishes with age, but the number of follicles is variable for every woman. A younger woman may have a lower number of antral follicles but the quality is still good versus an older woman with a high number of eggs but poor egg quality.

These two ultrasound images demonstrate normal ovarian reserve. The ovary size is appropriate; 12 follicles were counted on the right ovary, and 13 follicles were counted on the left ovary, totaling AFC of 25 follicles.

Figure 1.1

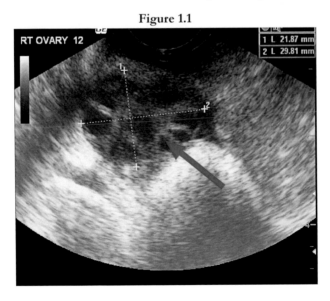

Figure 1.2

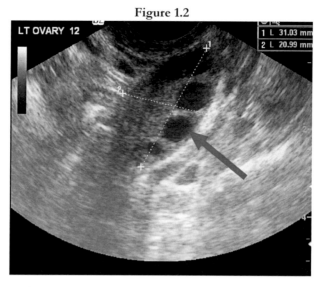

These ultrasound images demonstrate significant decrease in ovarian reserve. Often, the ovary may be smaller in size. Note that there is only 1 small black dot (antral follicle) noted on each ovary. This indicates that the egg supply is very low, so response of ovarian stimulation may be limited.

Figure 1.3

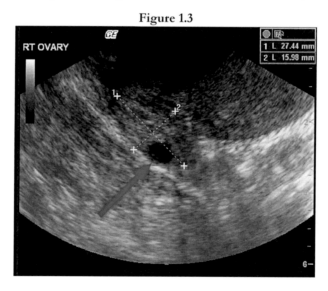

Figure 1.4

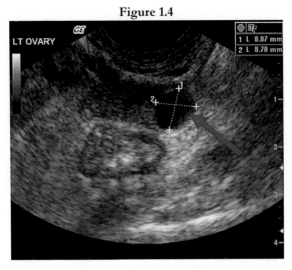

On these ultrasounds, over 30 antral follicles were counted on each ovary, and the ovary size is enlarged. This tells us that many follicles are present; this person may be at risk for over- responding to medications (ovarian hyperstimulation). The AFC helps determine the best dose of medication and treatment plan. An ovary with this many follicles may also point to polycystic ovarian syndrome (PCOS).

Figure 1.5

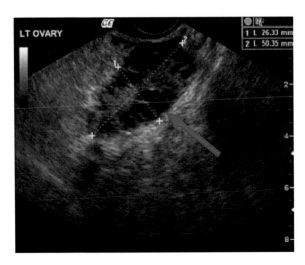

Figure 1.6

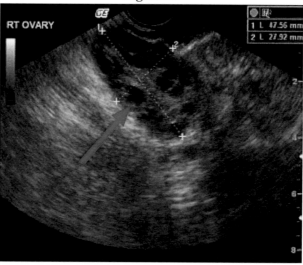

2. Semen analysis - the male evaluation

The semen analysis is the gold standard for the male evaluation. This test can tell if sperm are present, how many, and if they are moving. The semen analysis is important even if the male partner has previously fathered children. It can change during the reproductive years, but unlike eggs, sperm do not have a limited supply and new sperm are constantly being generated. If a semen analysis is abnormal, it should be repeated to confirm since values can frequently fluctuate. However, persistent abnormalities may require further consultation with a male fertility specialist (urologist).

For the semen analysis, it is recommended to have 2-3 days of abstinence, but not more than 10 days. Longer or shorter periods of abstinence may actually decrease a sperm count or motility. Men should also avoid hot tubs or saunas for at least 3 weeks prior to the test. I have seen totally normal sperm counts temporarily go to zero after using a hot tub because the heat destroyed the sperm.

TRAILHEAD TIP:

Any lubricants can cause a decline in sperm motility. Some manufacturers may state that they are "sperm friendly" which is better but can still cause a small decrease in motility.

There is also a misperception that men should "store up" their sperm prior to their partner's ovulation by abstaining from intercourse. Long periods of sexual inactivity actually results in more dead sperm and a decrease in their motility. For natural pregnancy attempts, intercourse every other day or every day is fine. There is no such thing as storing up sperm. Data shows that the highest chance of pregnancy is having intercourse before ovulation. Therefore, having frequent intercourse will help ensure that sperm will be ready and waiting in the fallopian tubes at the time of ovulation. In general, timed intercourse every day or every other day starting at least 6 days prior to ovulation is encouraged.

Often male patients ask me if there is anything they can take to improve their sperm quality. Some vitamin supplements may help although the data is inconclusive. Over-the-counter anti-oxidants supplements, such as Vitamin C (1000 mg per day) and Vitamin E (400 IU per day) may help with sperm quality.

You should talk to your provider regarding any medications that you are taking, including over-the-counter medications and supplements. For example, testosterone and steroids are especially detrimental to sperm production. Smoking and heavy alcohol use may also negatively impact sperm quality.

3. Tubal and uterine evaluation (if currently attempting pregnancy)

The fallopian tubes are critical for pregnancy to occur since this is where fertilization takes place. The test used to evaluate the fallopian tubes is called a hysterosalpingogram (HSG), which is an x-ray test. A contrast is slowly injected into the uterus while taking images. This test can tell us if your fallopian tubes are open or blocked or if there are any abnormalities.

The uterine cavity is the site where implantation occurs and the baby begins to grow. Therefore, it is good to evaluate the uterus for any abnormalities. We can see the uterine cavity during the HSG procedure and if there are any suspicions for an abnormality, another uterine evaluation test is often recommended. An office hysteroscopy (OH) or saline sonohysterogram (SIS) are procedures that look at the uterine cavity. Saline (like water) is infused into the uterus to visualize the uterine cavity with either with a small camera or ultrasound. These tests are typically done between days 5-12 of your menstrual cycle (when your period is over but before ovulation).

I have had these procedures and they do cause your uterus to cramp, like a bad menstrual period. If you don't have any allergies, I recommend taking a nonsteroidal anti-inflammatory (NSAID) medication such as Advil or Ibuprofen at least 1 hour prior to your procedure.

Normal hysterosalpingogram image showing the uterus and spill of dye into the pelvis.

Figure 1.7

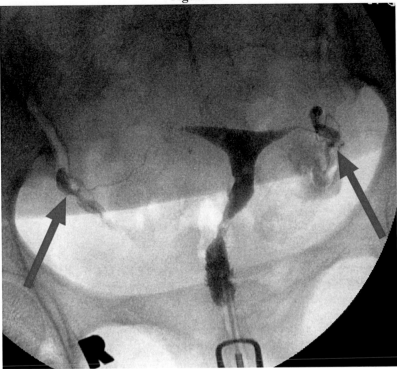

This is a saline sonohysterogram in which a polyp was found in the uterine cavity.

Figure 1.8

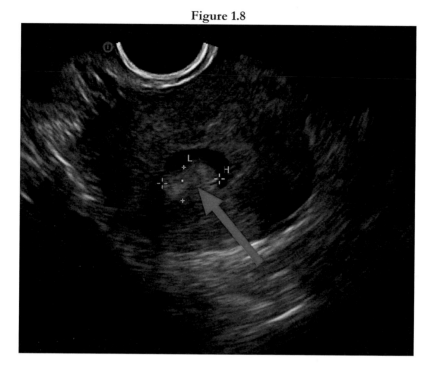

What can I do now to prepare my body for pregnancy?

This next section briefly reviews basic preconception health recommendations. I know there is a lot of this information widely available to you on the Internet; however, there are many myths or fad diets that quickly spread on social media, and I've been asked everything from eating pineapple to help with implantation to eating oysters to stimulate arousal.

The bottom line is to be healthy as best as you can. Eat a nutritious, balanced diet, and simply take care of yourself both physically and emotionally. Even when we do everything right, unforeseen events still can happen. I can be a perfectionist at times and in preparation for my own IVF cycle, I thought I did everything right. I took my prenatal vitamin daily for YEARS, limited my caffeine, and eliminated all alcohol use. I had enjoyed my glass of red wine with dinners, but having a healthy pregnancy was so important to me. Despite all of this, one of my sons was born with a cleft-lip and palate. This was not in our family history, and the reason for his congenital defect is thought to be multi-factorial. We also thought that he would be a vanishing twin because he was so small. This is my ultrasound image at 7 weeks of my pregnancy. You can easily see Twin 1 (labeled below) and then another tiny little black dot at the bottom of this image. That is twin B, our son, Jacob.

Figure 1.9

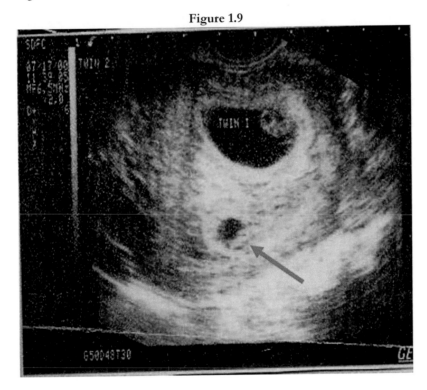

Annual examination, Pap smear, mammogram

Good health care starts with an annual exam, a Pap smear and a mammogram (if indicated) by your general OB/GYN provider. Completing this prior to pregnancy will also help facilitate the transition back to your OB provider once you are pregnant since you would already be an established patient.

Genetic testing

You or your partner (if applicable) may be a carrier of a genetic mutation that could affect your child(ren). Even though you may not have any signs or symptoms of disease, and there is none noted in your family history, routine genetic screening for at least one partner, prior to attempting pregnancy, is highly recommended and is really standard of care now.

Vaccinations

Diseases such as rubella, chicken pox, and seasonal flu can have serious implications during pregnancy and can be prevented with immunization. Even though most of us have probably been vaccinated, it does not mean you have immunity to the disease. Therefore, it is important to check your titer levels to see if you are immune or if you need to get a booster vaccination prior to pregnancy. I also recommend getting your flu shot every year which is safe while trying to get pregnant.

Chronic disease

Let your provider know about any chronic disease you may have, such as diabetes, seizure disorder, or high blood pressure. They may advise you to see a high-risk OB specialist (perinatologist) to help manage your care in order to optimize fertility and your pregnancy.

Medications

You will want to let your provider know of ALL medications or supplements you are taking. Your medications may need to be adjusted before pregnancy. Also, since herbal supplements are not regulated, I generally discourage them as well as many fertility providers.

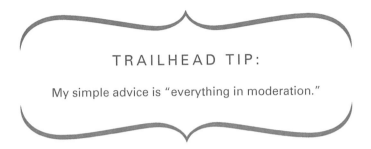

TRAILHEAD TIP:

My simple advice is "everything in moderation."

Mental health

I strongly encourage you to take care of yourself emotionally. This is much easier to say then do, but I truly believe this is important. Stress, depression, and anxiety are common consequences of infertility, and, trust me; I went through all of these. Try to find a healthy outlet if possible. Support groups may be helpful or talking with a fertility counselor. My mental health break was going for a walk and this continues to be my outlet.

Weight

A healthy weight is optimal, and many online BMI calculators may be used to learn your ideal weight for your height. If you are too thin or weigh too much, it can interrupt your menstrual cycles. Success rates are lower with obesity and there is an increased risk of complications such as gestational diabetes.

Exercise

"Is it ok to exercise?" The answer in general is "yes." Exercise is a healthy activity and can make you feel better. I love to walk and get fresh air; I use it as my stress relief. However, strenuous activity that involves bouncing or jarring the ovaries should be avoided during ovarian stimulation when your ovaries may become enlarged. Too much exercise may also interfere with ovulation. The key is moderation.

Quit smoking and avoid or limit alcohol

Smoking has been shown to negatively impact both egg and sperm quality. Alcohol should be avoided or limited to no more than 1-2 drinks per week, and none after ovulation, intrauterine insemination, or embryo transfer. Yes, you can have a glass of wine with dinner in the early part of your menstrual cycle, but after ovulation or embryo transfer, you will want to treat your body as if you are pregnant, and alcohol is not safe during pregnancy.

Diet

A nutritious, balanced diet with lots of fruits, vegetables, protein, and whole grains are always best. Try to avoid processed foods, fast foods, and sodas containing empty nutrients.

Eating healthy now will set the stage for healthy eating during pregnancy and hopefully through your life. However, do not worry if you have a few must-have cravings. My craving was ice cream! My favorite was vanilla ice cream mixed with 2 tablespoons of peanut butter and 2 teaspoons of chocolate milk power. Yum!

Prenatal Vitamin

Taking a daily prenatal vitamin is sufficient whether you are freezing eggs or attempting pregnancy. Look for a trusted prenatal vitamin with a certified or verified label and one that contains 800-1000 mcg folic acid, Vitamin D, at least 150 mcg iodine, and 200mg DHA.

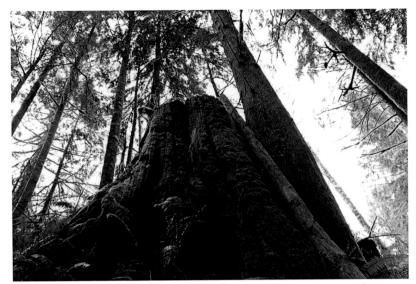

No stump can get in your way; instead open your arms around it.

Rest stop to regroup

We're off to a great start on our fertility walk! Together we've covered the initial consultation, the follow up, fertility evaluation basics, and tips for preparing your body for pregnancy. I encourage you to take some time to consolidate your information and questions here so you're ready for the next leg of our journey: Female Anatomy and Your Monthly Cycle.

What are the good things you are doing right now to prepare for pregnancy?

What are some things you could improve?

What questions do you have for your provider?

Notes:

http://www.davidalbeck.com/hiking/glossary.html; June 17, 2015

Chapter 2

Female Anatomy

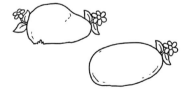

Female Anatomy

Orienteering: (verb) - A trek using a map and compass to find one's way through unfamiliar territory.[i]

Bearing: **(noun)** - A specific direction, typically with an assigned degree, usually used when navigating with a compass.[ii]

Thinking back to my experience as a patient, I remember the confusion I felt as I looked at my ultrasound and tried to understand the image before me. Now as a provider, I appreciate how difficult it may be for my patients as well. This chapter devoted to female anatomy and ultrasound will better equip you for just such a scenario. I want you to feel confident and empowered to understand your own ultrasound and be able to ask questions along the way. Instead of a map and a compass, we'll use physiology to find our way through the unfamiliar territory of the female anatomy.

As I mentioned earlier, transvaginal ultrasound is a valuable tool in the evaluation and management of fertility and early pregnancy. Ultrasound uses high frequency sound waves given off by the transducer to create images you can see on the ultrasound screen, and is perfectly safe. We will review some actual ultrasound images in this book and help explain what they mean.

Figure 2.1 Uterus in long axis view

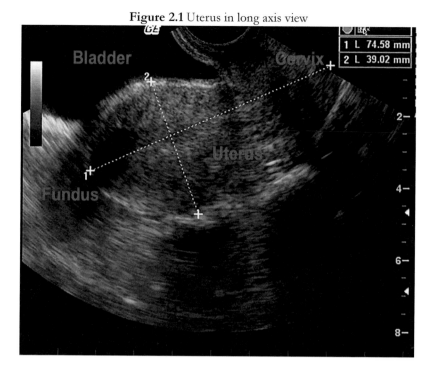

The diagram above illustrates the uterus, cervix, fundus (or top of the uterus) and the bladder. The cervix is approximately 3-5 centimeters in length and can easily be seen on ultrasound. The cervix is the canal opening up into the uterine cavity. Some women may have a sharp bend in their cervix (illustration below shows a cervix with a sharp bend). This bend may sometimes make intrauterine inseminations (IUI) or embryo transfer a bit tricky.

TRAILHEAD TIP:

Your provider may recommend a partial to full bladder prior to your IUI or embryo transfer procedure in order to help straighten the cervix and allow easier transfer of the catheter into the uterus.

Figure 2.2 Cervix with sharp bend

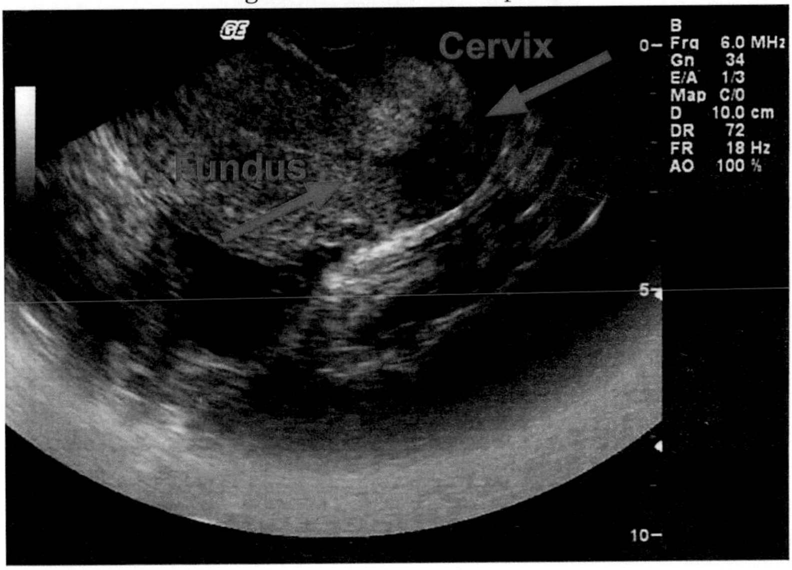

The Uterus

Visually, many people describe the uterus like the size of a pear. The uterus can be in several different positions based on normal anatomy and every woman's anatomy is unique. Uterine position does not influence your chance of getting pregnant. It may, however, present difficulties during the following procedures: ultrasound imaging, IUI, and embryo transfer.

The uterine position is described according to the fundus (or top of the uterus) and its position relative to the cervix. In an anteverted uterus, the fundus is pointing forward relative to the cervix. A retroverted uterus is when the fundus is pointing backwards. A woman with a retroverted uterus may also experience more back pain with her menstrual cycles and ovulation. Of note, the uterine position can be influenced by fullness of the bladder.

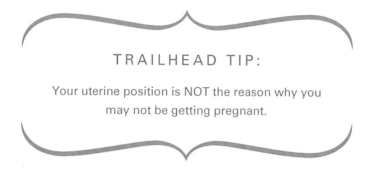

TRAILHEAD TIP:

Your uterine position is NOT the reason why you
may not be getting pregnant.

Figure 2.3 Anteverted uterine position

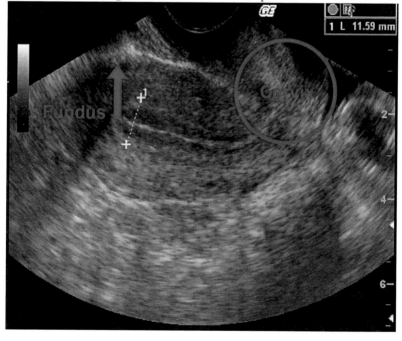

Figure 2.4 Retroverted uterine position

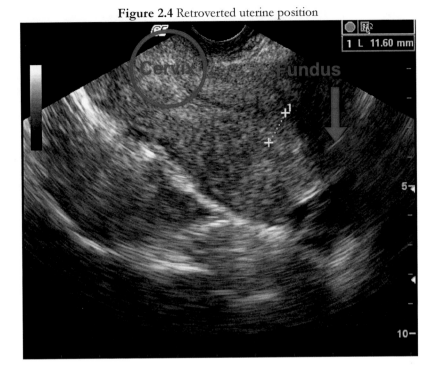

Fallopian Tubes

The fallopian tubes are very thin, often described like spaghetti noodles, and are usually not seen on ultrasound unless they contain fluid or are surrounded by fluid, indicating an abnormal finding.

The fallopian tube is where fertilization naturally occurs; therefore a normal, functioning tube is critical for fertilization. If one or both fallopian tubes are blocked or not functioning appropriately, then in-vitro fertilization (IVF) may be advised.

During an IUI, the sperm sample is deposited into the uterus, and then the sperm swim up into both fallopian tubes. Sperm are actually attracted towards the egg. The pinpoint opening into the fallopian tubes is so small it can only be visualized with a specialized camera called a hysteroscope.

The sausage looking area on the ultrasound image shown here is a dilated fallopian tube. Seeing a fallopian tube on ultrasound is an abnormal finding (see chapter 4, hydrosalpinx).

Figure 2.5 Fallopian tube filled with fluid

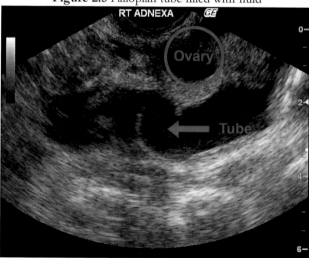

Endometrium

The endometrium is viewed as a separate entity within the uterus. This is where implantation occurs and where the embryo begins to grow. The endometrium is composed of a basal and functional layer. The basal layer is permanent while the functional layer is the layer that responds to monthly hormonal changes in the menstrual cycle. The functional layer shedding is called menses or a period. During menses, your endometrium is typically thin. It will then begin to thicken as estrogen increases from the follicle (egg) growing. Your provider will measure your endometrial thickness on ultrasound to ensure that it is adequate to maintain a pregnancy.

Too thick or too thin? The most common endometrial measurements are between 8-13 millimeters. A thin lining, < 6 millimeters, may be concerning for implantation and may be a result of uterine scarring or adhesions. A thick lining, > 15-16 millimeters may result from a polyp or fibroid and further evaluation may be warranted.

Figure 2.6 Endometrium in long axis

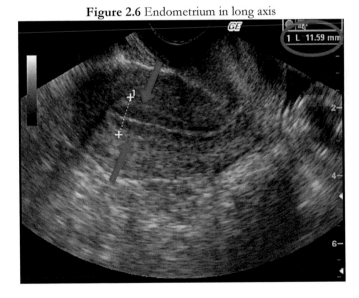

Ovaries

The ovaries are normally about the size of an almond. They are usually located on either side of uterus and are held by ligaments. The ovaries respond to hormonal changes in the menstrual cycle. Typically during the reproductive years, the female ovary contains several antral follicles that can be seen on ultrasound. These tiny follicles can be counted to give us a general idea of your egg supply (the AFC evaluation). In women with regular menstrual cycles each month, one follicle will grow to become the dominant follicle that will ovulate, and the other follicles will die. The hormone, luteinizing hormone (LH), initiates ovulation during which time the egg is released. At ovulation, the mature egg will reduce its number of chromosomes by one-half so it is ready for the sperm's chromosomes to fertilize the other half.

This is a normal looking ovary on ultrasound. The black dots are antral follicles.

Figure 2.7 Normal ovary with antral follicles

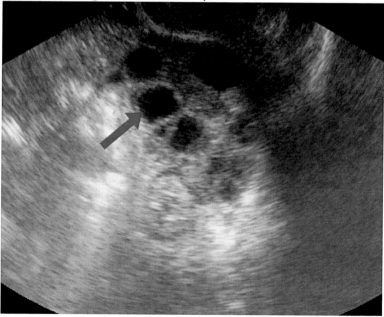

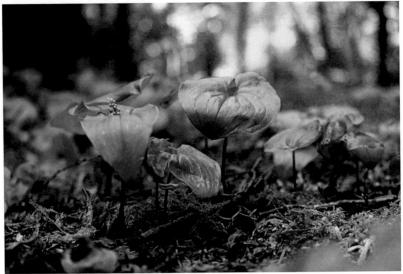

Delicate soft whisperings makes each of us unique.

Rest stop to regroup

Some women embark on their fertility walk and become overwhelmed right at the outset. The unfamiliarity of medical terms and seemingly invasive procedures can discourage even the most determined patients. I've thrown a lot of terms and images at you in this chapter. Take a minute to write down your own questions, concerns, and notes on the topic of female anatomy and ultrasounds.

Questions for your provider:

Notes:

http://hike-nh.com/faq/glossary/; June 17, 2015

http://hike-nh.com/faq/glossary/; June 19, 2015

Chapter 3

Understanding The Menstrual Cycle

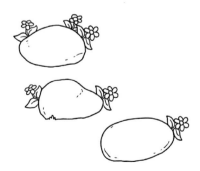

Understanding The Menstrual Cycle

Scramble: (verb) - Typically refers to the act of climbing over rock fields or rough terrain.[i]

Cairn: (noun) - The stone piles often erected along a trail above tree line, to serve as an indicator of trail direction.[ii]

This next section will review the menstrual cycle with ultrasound images to help further explain the normal reproductive system. For the non-medically inclined, this can be a bit of a hike over rough terrain. Hang in there; although sometimes difficult to maneuver at times, the science behind infertility will greatly assist you through this journey. The female reproductive system is truly fascinating and unlike any other organ in the body, the pelvic structures undergo cyclic, physiologic changes that can be observed and followed on ultrasound.

The menstrual cycle is divided into four stages: the menses, follicular or proliferative, ovulation, and the luteal or secretory phase. I have described each phase below with an example of what is happening in the uterus as well as in the ovaries. The ultrasound illustrations further explain this normal physiologic process and gives you a visual.

Figure 3.1

Phase	Cycle Days
Menstrual	1 - 4
Follicular or Proliferative	5 - 13
Ovulation	~14~
Luteal or Secretory	15 - 28

Phase 1: The Menstrual Cycle or Menses

Phase 1 is when a woman is on her period (aka menstrual cycle).

The uterus in phase one

The endometrium is the lining of the uterus. On the menses (your period) the endometrium appears as a thin line because the functional layer was shed as described in chapter 2. For most women, the average length of the period is 2-7 days with the heaviest flow in the first 2 days.

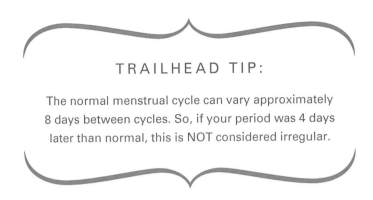

TRAILHEAD TIP:

The normal menstrual cycle can vary approximately
8 days between cycles. So, if your period was 4 days
later than normal, this is NOT considered irregular.

The following is an ultrasound image during the menses. You can see the thin endometrial line referred to as the "stripe."

Figure 3.2 Thin endometrium on menses

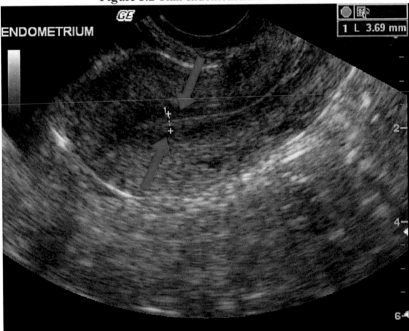

Ultrasound image of the endometrium on cycle day 5 of the menses (period). The lining is slightly thicker, now close to 6 millimeters.

Figure 3.3

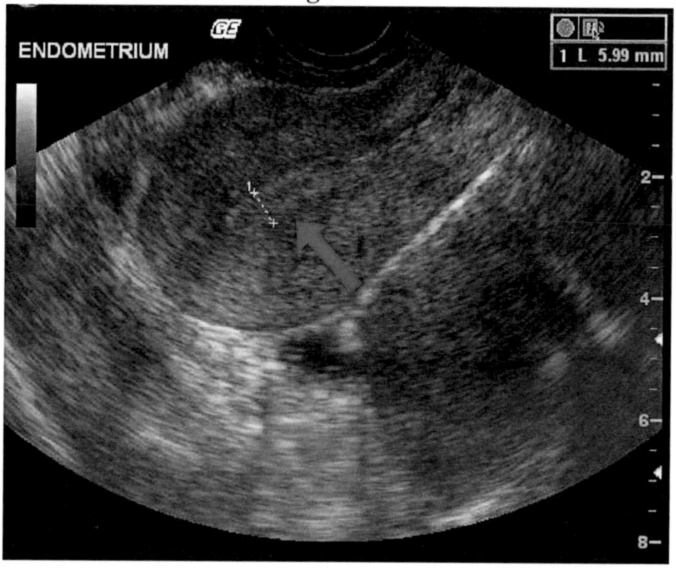

The ovary in phase 1

The normal ovary contains several antral follicles that can be seen on ultra-sound. Antral follicles are the "selectable" follicles. As I mentioned earlier, I call them the little wannabes. From these several antral follicles, one will become the dominant follicle that will go on to ovulate. The other small follicles will die back, which is referred to as atresia. Atresia is a normal degenerative process that occurs regardless of whether you have normal menstrual cycles, use birth control pills, are pregnant, or undergoing infertility treatment. At puberty you have about 180,000-300,000 eggs and around age 42, it is down to approximately 1000 eggs. Out of hundreds of thousands of eggs, only around 300 eggs will ovulate during your entire reproductive years; the rest will die back.

An ultrasound image of a normal size ovary with antral follicles.

Figure 3.4 Normal ovary

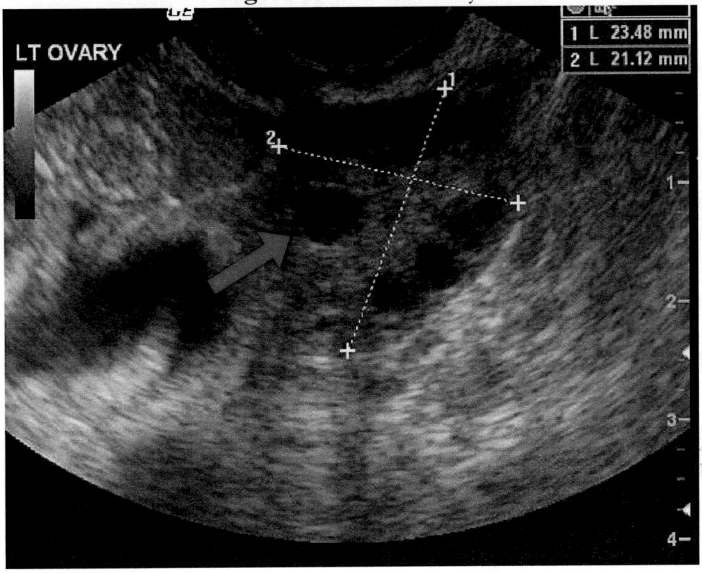

Phase 2: The Proliferative and Follicular Phase

The uterus in phase 2

The proliferative phase refers to the development of the endometrial lining. This phase occurs between days 5-13 of the menstrual cycle when the endometrium begins to thicken. On ultrasound, the multilayer or 3 line pattern forms from the glands. The outer line is the interface between endometrium and myometrium (the uterine muscle), and the inner line represents the swelling of the functional layer from estrogen that is being secreted from the developing follicle (egg).

As the follicle grows, the endometrium also grows in response to the increase in estradiol (estrogen) released from the developing egg. The growth of the endometrium may reach a maximum between 8-16 millimeters. There is often an increase in cervical mucus experienced by some women as they get closer to ovulation. This increase in cervical mucus results from rising levels of estrogen.

The endometrium in this ultrasound image is thicker now, 11.6 millimeters, and the pattern has changed to what is commonly called "trilaminar" or "triple line" in appearance.

Figure 3.5 Endometrium in the proliferative phase

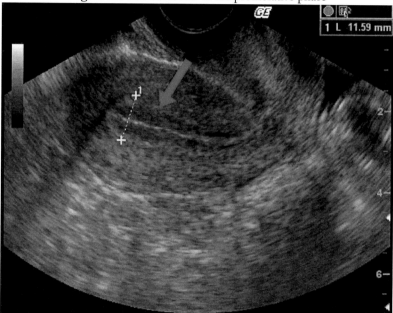

The Ovary in Phase 2

The follicular phase refers to the development of the dominant follicle (egg). Granulosa cells in the developing follicle secrete estrogen and follicular fluid. An ultrasound reveals this phase with an increase of the follicle size. In a normal menstrual cycle (without any stimulation medications), one follicle will become the lead or dominant follicle while the others will digress.

Under ovarian stimulation with oral ovulation medications, the average number of mature follicles is 1-2 follicles. Several follicles may start to grow, but often most of them will not pass 10-14 millimeters in size before degenerating. Our goal as fertility providers is to either achieve ovulation with one dominant follicle or to superovulate with 2-3 mature follicles. More than 3 follicles increases your chance of high order multiple pregnancy.

The dominant follicle grows approximately 2 millimeters per day and will usually emerge around day 8-12 of the menstrual cycle. This is why many fertility providers recommend an ultrasound around days 10-12 of the menstrual cycle to evaluate your ovulatory pattern or to assess your response to oral ovulation induction medications. These ultrasound images show the growth of a dominant follicle in a normal menstrual cycle.

Figure 3.6 Cycle day 5 - normal ovary

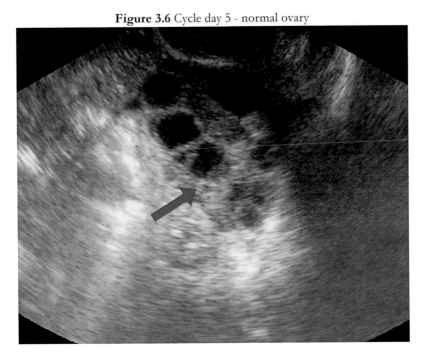

Figure 3.7 Cycle day 8 - The dominant follicle has emerged; average size is 12.5 millimeters

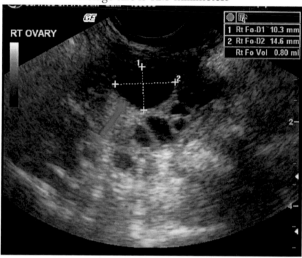

Figure 3.8 Cycle day 11 - The dominant follicle is growing, sized at 17 millimeters

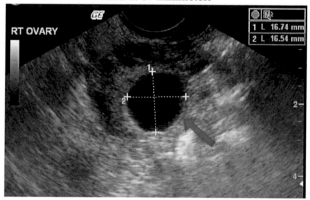

Figure 3.9 Cycle Day 15 – The dominant follicle is mature and ready to ovulate; size is now 25 millimeters

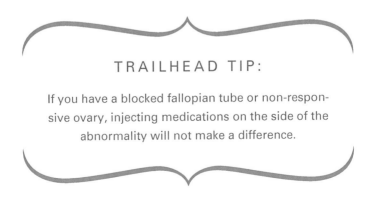

Phase 3: Ovulation

A dominant or mature follicle can measure between 13-33 millimeters, quite a wide range. I often get asked how do I know the egg is mature. Although eggs are microscopic, we can measure the follicle (fluid surrounding the egg) on ultrasound. The most common size of a mature follicle is 20-25 mm; if the follicle measures this size and the endometrium also looks appropriately thick, we can assume the egg is mature and close to ovulation.

TRAILHEAD TIP:

If you have a blocked fallopian tube or non-responsive ovary, injecting medications on the side of the abnormality will not make a difference.

The side of the dominant follicle is random; a woman may ovulate from the right ovary 2-3 months in a row, which can be very frustrating if that is the side of a blocked fallopian tube. Hormonally, the normal mid-cycle estrogen level is approximately 200 pg/mL (range 100-300 pg/mL). This rise in estrogen level from the growing follicle stimulates the luteinizing hormone (LH) surge.

This ultrasound image reflects a dominant, mature follicle and measures 20.5 millimeters.

Figure 3.10 Possible cumulous oophorus with impending ovulation

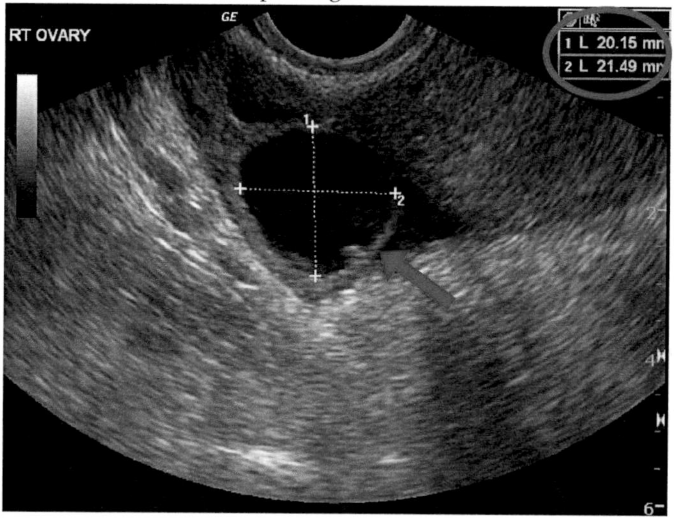

TRAILHEAD TIP:

The LH surge is really variable and the duration is not always 3 days. Some women may peak and only have one day when they see the positive.

Assessment of ovulation

There are several ways to assess ovulation, described below. These include Basal Body Temperature (BBT), Ovulation Predictor Kits (OPKs), and a progesterone blood test.

Basal body temperature (BBT)

Many online tools are available to assist you with basal body temperature charting. In short, you take your basal body temperature daily and graph the results. In a normal ovulatory cycle, the graph should demonstrate a low then higher pattern, referred to as a biphasic pattern. This pattern simply correlates with ovulation. The BBT chart may be initially useful for your provider to see if you have ovulatory patterns, however BBT charting is NOT useful for predicting the day of ovulation or timing intercourse. Charting for 2-3 months should be enough to see if you have a cyclic pattern or not. I do not recommend testing any longer. I did it for over 1 year and it became a constant reminder that I was not pregnant.

Figure 3.11

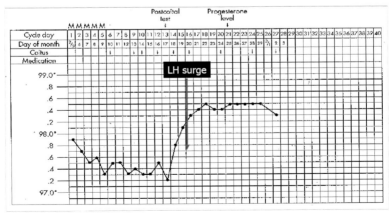

Ovulation predictor kits (OPKs)

Ovulation predictor kits measure the amount of urinary luteinizing hormone (LH) as a marker of ovulation. LH increases before ovulation, commonly called "LH surge." The day you start OPKs may vary depending on your menstrual cycle length. For example, if you have a 28-day cycle, it is often recommended to start urine LH testing on cycle day 11. I recommend talking to your provider, nurse, or coordinator regarding what day you should start testing based on your medical history. You don't want to waste several test strips because you started too early or miss your surge because you started too late.

The LH surge lasts 48-58 hours and the egg will ovulate 34-36 hours after the onset of the LH surge. The majority of women begin their LH surge between midnight and 8 a.m. The OPK manufacturer may recommend first-void morning testing, but afternoon testing is fine as well. Testing in the afternoon may help with early detection of your surge onset rather than waiting until the following morning when it will also be positive.

There are two main types of ovulation predictor kits. One type uses a test strip, which is compared to the reference line; another type, referred to as "digital," shows a smiley face or "YES" in the test window.

On any given day, I get more questions about ovulation kits than anything else. They can sometimes by quite frustrating and give confusing results. Some couples find them particularly stressful, and intercourse can become dictated by time. I hope you will find these tips useful:

- You do not need to hold your urine for 4 hours prior to testing.
- If using test strips, a positive is when the color is equal or darker than the reference line.
- The manufacturer states the color needs to be darker than the reference, but if it is equal, it is considered a positive.
- OPKs DO NOT work with all women. Do not get frustrated or disappointed if you do not get a positive on the kit. We have many alternative ways to induce ovulation.

- OPKs can be confusing to use; I found they weren't worth the time and stress, and I eventually stopped using them.

- You do not need to test your urine more than once a day. In fact, we discourage it.

- Cycles can vary, and you may not get your LH surge on the same day every month, which is normal.

- OPKs test the signal to ovulate from the brain and NOT when actual ovulation occurs. When an OPK is positive, it means that ovulation will occur approximately within the next 36 hours.

Intercourse or insemination timing

- Do not stress over timing, it's not exact.

- Regular intercourse is encouraged, preferably daily or every other day as ovulation approaches. One is not better than the other.

- There is no such thing as "storing up" sperm. In fact, abstaining more than 5 days may decrease sperm quality.

- If timing of intercourse feels too demanding, don't worry. Timed intercourse once or twice is sufficient.

- Inseminations are generally performed 20-36 hours following a positive OPK.

- If given a hCG injection "trigger shot," inseminations are timed approximately 24-38 hours after the injection.

- If given a hCG injection for timed intercourse, start having intercourse the day of hCG trigger and then every day or every other day for the next 5-6 days.

Progesterone blood test

Progesterone is secreted after ovulation and can be measured in a blood test. Levels can fluctuate, and if your cycle length is long or variable, a single level (often referred to as a "day 21 progesterone level") may not be accurate. If performing a single blood test, it is better to do the blood test one week after a positive result on an ovulation predictor kit. Some providers may perform multiple blood progesterone blood tests after ovulation and then average the results; this is referred to as "pooled progesterone testing." The pooled test may be more representative of the entire luteal phase.

The following images on ultrasound reflect recent ovulation. The dominant follicle may look irregular or deflated on ultrasound at the time of ovulation. You may sometimes see free fluid in the cul-de-sac on ultrasound just after ovulation. As the follicle ruptured, follicular fluid was released and the egg was expelled.

Figure 3.12 Irregular deflated follicle on ultrasound

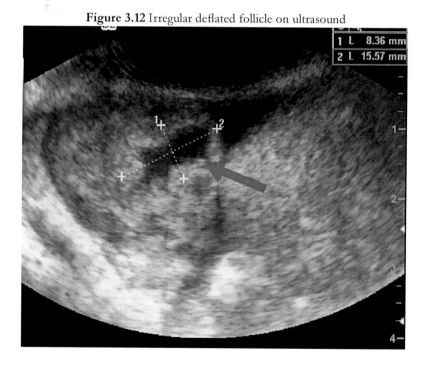

Figure 3.13 Free fluid noted consistent with ovulation

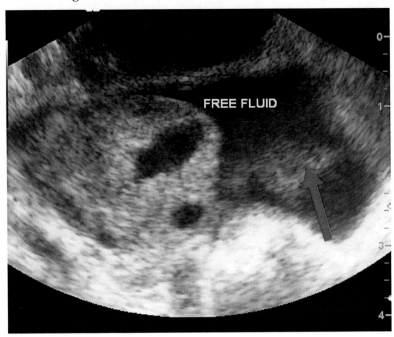

Phase 4: Luteal Phase — Ovary

The ovary in phase 4

After ovulation, the follicle that contained the egg develops into a corpus luteum cyst. The corpus luteum secrets progesterone to help support an early pregnancy. If there is no pregnancy, the corpus luteum will digress, progesterone levels will drop, and a menstrual cycle or period will start.

This ultrasound image is a corpus luteum cyst seen right after ovulation. Note the internal echoes, which are strands from a blood clot.

Figure 3.14 Fresh corpus luteum

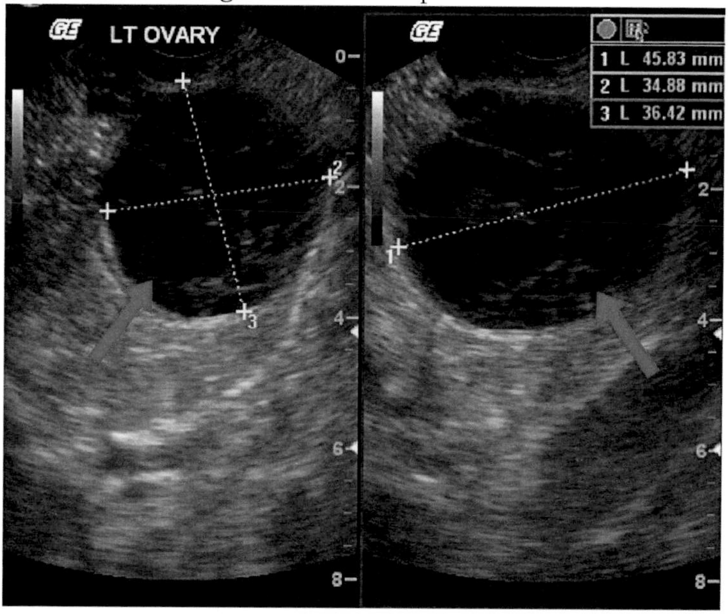

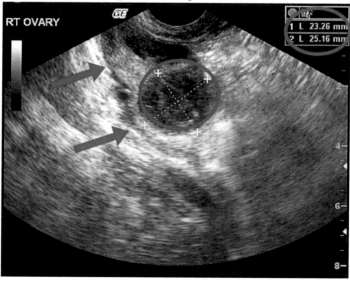

As mentioned above, the corpus luteum develops after ovulation. The average size is 2.5 – 3 centimeters. They can sometimes get larger if blood is leaking into the cyst.

Figure 3.15 Corpus Luteum

Ultrasound images of the corpus luteal cyst. Again, these types of cysts are part of normal ovulatory function.

Figure 3.16

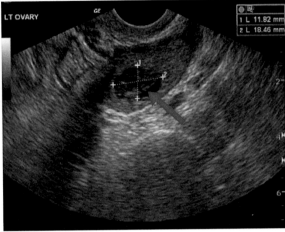

Phase 4: Secretory Phase — Uterus

The uterus in phase 4

After ovulation, progesterone causes the endometrium to look solid or homogeneous on ultrasound. There is no longer the 3 line pattern as described in the proliferative phase earlier.

Figure 3.17 Luteal phase endometrium

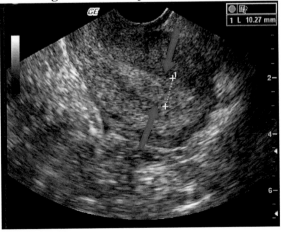

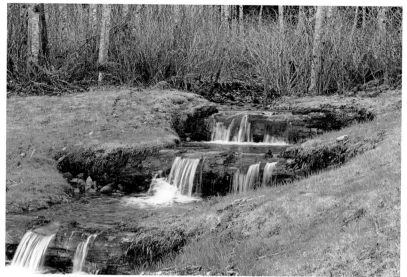

You can take a walk in nature to understand nature.

Rest stop to regroup

Okay, go ahead and stop to catch your breath. The last thing I want is to send you into overload paralysis. To summarize, the normal reproductive cycle is divided into 4 phases:

Phase 1: The menstrual cycle or menses
Phase 2: The proliferative and follicular phase
Phase 3: Ovulation
Phase 4: Luteal and Secretory Phase

Your fertility provider is an expert on these 4 cycles as well as on techniques/procedures to try depending on your particular menstrual cycle. Remember, you are not alone in your journey; you might be surprised when you realize how many women struggle through the "natural" process of conception. Keep reading, keep learning, keep asking questions.

Questions for your provider:

Notes:

http://hike-nh.com/faq/glossary/; June 20, 2015

ibid

Chapter 4

A Look at
Cysts, Polyps, Fibroids, and
Other Abnormalities

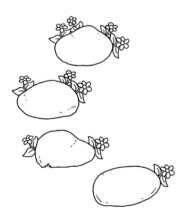

A Look at Cysts, Fibroids, Polyps, and Other Abnormalities

Self-arrest: (verb) – The act of halting one's own descent, as when sliding downslope. Not as easy as it sounds.[i]

Switchback: (noun) – A trail that travels diagonally and turns back on itself in order to allow progression up a steep section of a mountain.[ii]

After your ultrasound, your provider may discuss the findings of a cyst or fibroid. Although these are very common findings in reproductive medicine, this information may be concerning and even overwhelming; you may feel like a hiker who's just lost footing on a steep incline. As a medical provider, I see cysts and fibroids almost every day. I hope this chapter will reassure and help you understand your ultrasound findings, and offer you explanations. You may discover this news may reveal itself to be less about sliding downhill and more like a switchback; you're still progressing up the path towards fertility, it just feels like you're going in reverse.

Ovarian cysts

During the course of a lifetime, many women may develop an ovarian cyst. Most ovarian cysts are a part of normal ovarian function. However, a cyst that is present prior to starting fertility treatment could interfere with cycle timing. These cysts can understandably elicit anxiety and concern and are especially frustrating if they cause a delay in your treatment.

Ovarian cysts are often described as simple (cystic), complex, or solid. Additionally, they can be classified as functional versus nonfunctional. A functional cyst means that the granulosa cells within the follicle remain productive and they are secreting estrogen. This is why an estrogen blood test is often done when a new cyst has been identified on ultrasound. The estrogen blood test will help your provider determine if your cyst is functional or not. If your estrogen blood test is elevated (usually noted above 50 pg/mL), then your cycle may be postponed until the cyst resolves or your estrogen level drops. A hormonally active cyst may also cause your menstrual cycle to be irregular.

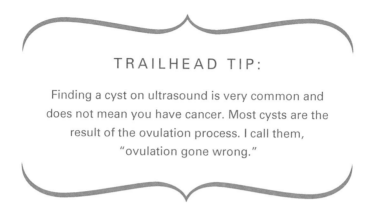

TRAILHEAD TIP:

Finding a cyst on ultrasound is very common and does not mean you have cancer. Most cysts are the result of the ovulation process. I call them, "ovulation gone wrong."

A nonfunctional cyst is described when the granulosa cells lose their ability to produce estrogen, and the estrogen blood test is low. In most cases, a nonfunctional cyst can be ignored, and treatment is often started depending on the size of the nonfunctional cyst.

Functional cysts are quite common and result from the normal ovulatory process. These are ovulation related cysts, meaning that they result from the nonrupture of a dominant follicle or failure of an immature follicle to undergo atresia (degeneration). For example, if you were on birth control pills for cycle coordination, the birth control pills should suppress ovulation. However, sometimes a follicle may try to develop but then it is suppressed. That follicle now has evolved into a cyst.

When a cyst is identified, it is usually recommended to have a follow-up ultrasound to document that the cyst has resolved or is stable.

Simple cysts

This is a simple cyst. An estrogen blood test would help classify if the cyst is functional or nonfunctional. In all of the examples, you can see that the cyst is fluid which appears black on ultrasound.

Figure 4.1

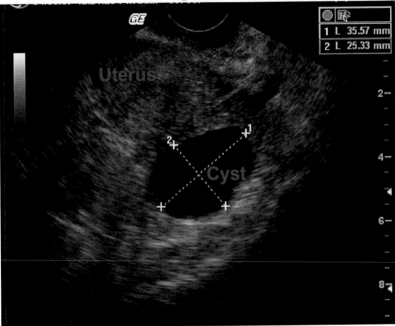

This simple cyst looks just like a developing follicle on ultrasound. This would be a normal finding on day 14 of your cycle, but if you are on your menses or period, there should not be any cysts or large looking follicles.

Figure 4.2

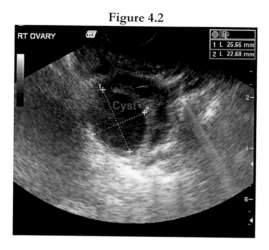

This is a large simple cyst. There are rare potential complications when a cyst is this large, such as rupture with bleeding or torsion (twisting of the ovarian ligament). The symptom would be pain. If you have a large cyst, you should call your provider if you experience any pain. It is also advised to limit physical activity, avoid heavy lifting >20 pounds, and be on pelvic rest (no intercourse) until the cyst resolves.

Figure 4.3

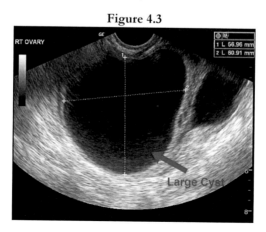

Paraovarian or paratubal cysts

Paraovarian or paratubal cysts look like a simple cyst, but they are located outside the ovary. This type of cyst is simply a fluid-filled sac and is presumed to be a remnant of your own fetal development. Most paraovarian cysts are small, and they do not have any symptoms or require any treatment. They will sometimes even disappear on their own. These cysts are really an incidental finding and have no impact on your fertility treatment.

This cyst looks like a simple cyst, but you can see that it is located outside the ovary.

Figure 4.4 Paraovarian or paratubal cyst

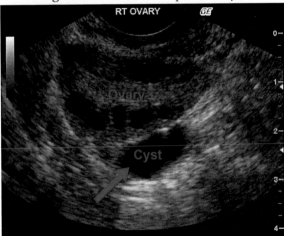

Complex cysts - corpus luteal cyst

The development of a corpus luteum cyst is a normal part of the ovulation process. If pregnancy does not occur, the corpus luteum will degenerate and will be gone by the start of the menses. A corpus luteum cyst can develop when the escape opening of the egg seals off and fluid or blood accumulates inside the follicle. In this case, the corpus luteum does not degenerate within the normal time frame and can persist, often causing the menstrual cycle to be irregular. Most corpus luteum cysts will spontaneously resolve within 6 to 12 weeks.

This type of cyst looks complex (different shadows of gray versus dark black as seen in a simple cyst). This would be a normal finding after ovulation, but this cyst should resolve by the time you start your menses or period.

Figure 4.5 Corpus luteum cyst

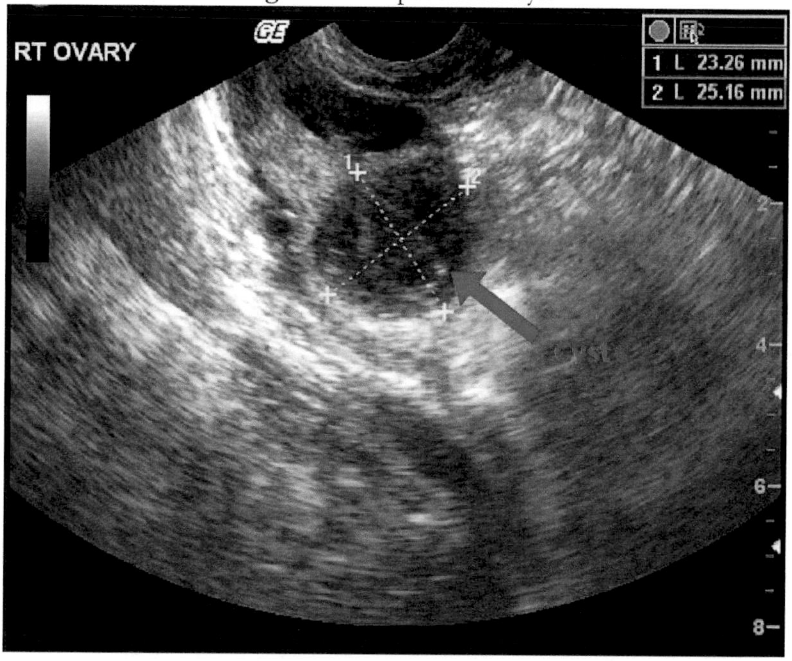

This cyst is also complex in appearance with white strands that look web-like. Those strands are the ultrasound image of the blood clot trapped in the corpus luteum. This type of cyst is often referred to as "hemorrhagic," meaning there is bleeding within the cyst.

Figure 4.6

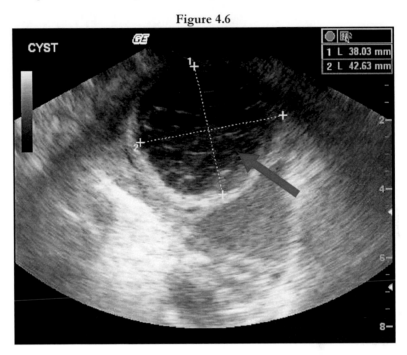

Complex cyst – endometrioma

Endometriosis occurs when cells in the endometrial tissue (lining of your uterus) travel outside the uterus and implant in other areas such as the ovary or pelvis. These cells respond to normal ovulation hormonal changes, and they bleed just like you bleed during your menses or period. The implantation of this endometrial tissue outside the uterus can cause symptoms such as pelvic pain, menstrual cramps, painful intercourse, and infertility. Additionally, the bleeding can cause local inflammation, which leads to the development of adhesions in the pelvis.

An endometrioma is a cyst on the ovary that is a result from the accumulation of cells and blood. Endometriomas are commonly found in reproductive medicine and see at least one endometrioma daily. Finding an endometrioma on ultrasound may help your provider explain your infertility. In general, complications from endometriomas are very rare. Endometriomas are described as a complex cyst, and they tend to have a classic dull gray or "ground glass" appearance. This type of cyst may have to be surgically removed depending on its size and symptoms.

Examples of endometriomas

Figure 4.7

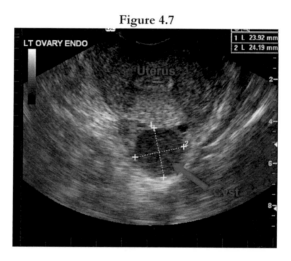

Figure 4.8

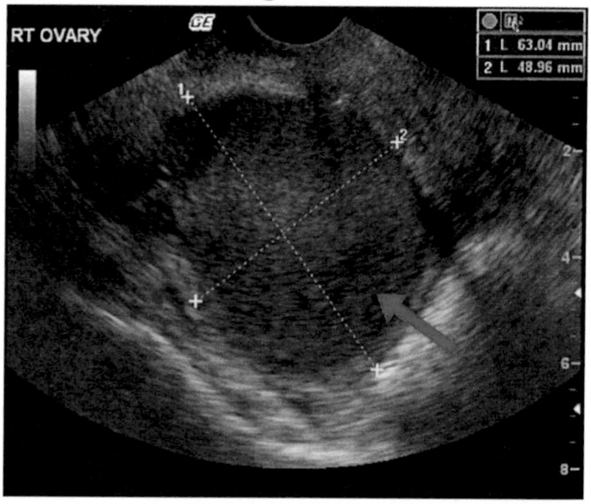

Figure 4.9 Endometrioma

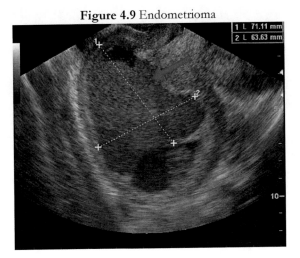

Complex cyst – dermoid

A dermoid is a benign cyst sometimes referred to as a cystic teratoma. Ovarian dermoid cysts originate from trapped germ cells that are present at birth. This type of cyst may contain other growths of body tissues, such as fat, bone, hair, and cartilage. Most dermoid cysts have no symptoms, and the chance of transforming into a cancerous lesion is rare. Uncommon complications may include infection if the cyst ruptures and ovarian torsion.

On ultrasound, a dermoid cyst is complex in appearance with several different echoes or shades of gray. The bright echoes are from calcifications, teeth, and bone.

Examples of a dermoid cyst

Figure 4.10

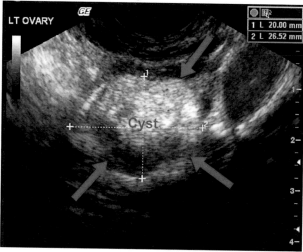

Figure 4.11

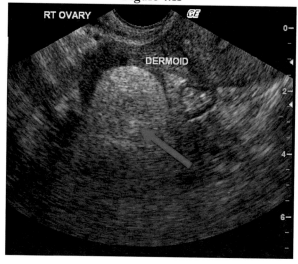

Solid mass

Fortunately, solid masses are not common in reproductive age women. However, if one is found, further testing and surgical intervention may be required.

In general, there is an increased risk of malignancy or cancer if the cyst is large (5-7 centimeters in diameter), complex, or solid in appearance, and persists over time. Symptoms of ovarian cancer may be vague and include back pain, abdominal bloating, gastrointestinal irritability, or pelvic pressure.

A cyst with the following characteristics will need to be further discussed and analyzed by your physician:

- The cyst wall is thick or irregular
- An increased and disorganized blood supply within the mass (blood supply is critical for cancer growth)
- The cyst size is large, greater than 7 centimeters
- The cyst has solid components, nodules, or papillary projections which can be seen within the cyst

Examples of concerning cysts found on ultrasound

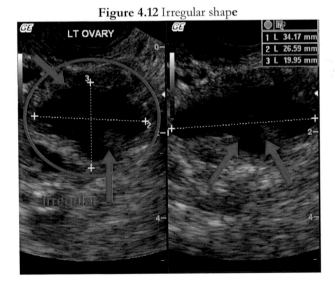

Figure 4.12 Irregular shape

Figure 4.13 Solid area within a large cyst

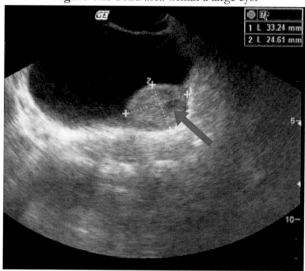

Figure 4.14 Multiple solid areas within a large cyst

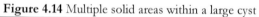

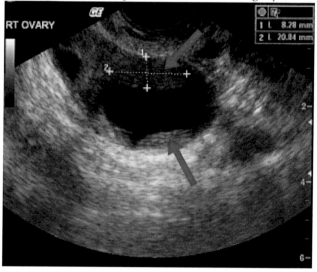

Uterine fibroids

Uterine fibroids are another very common finding in reproductive medicine. In fact, they occur in up to 30-40% in women older than 35 years of age. A fibroid is a non-cancerous (benign) tumor that is composed of smooth muscle cells that grow from the uterine muscle. A fibroid can cause your uterus to be enlarged or irregular. If a fibroid is distorting your uterine cavity or is located within the cavity, it may impact fertility and further evaluation may be warranted. Sometimes, surgically removing the fibroid may be recommended by your provider.

Fibroids are described by their location. Types of fibroids include the following:

- Subserosal – These fibroids are on the outside of the uterus
- Intramural – These are the most common type of fibroids and are located in the muscle of the uterus
- Submucosal – This type of fibroid is found within the uterine cavity or lining. They may impact fertility and because they are located in the endometrium can also cause heavy or prolonged bleeding during menses

The following ultrasound images are examples of uterine fibroids.

Figure 4.15

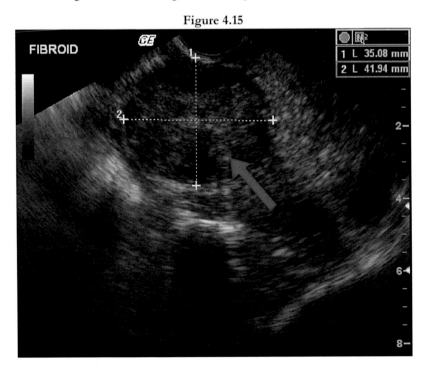

Subserosal – Fibroids outside of the uterus

Figure 4.16 Subserosal fibroid

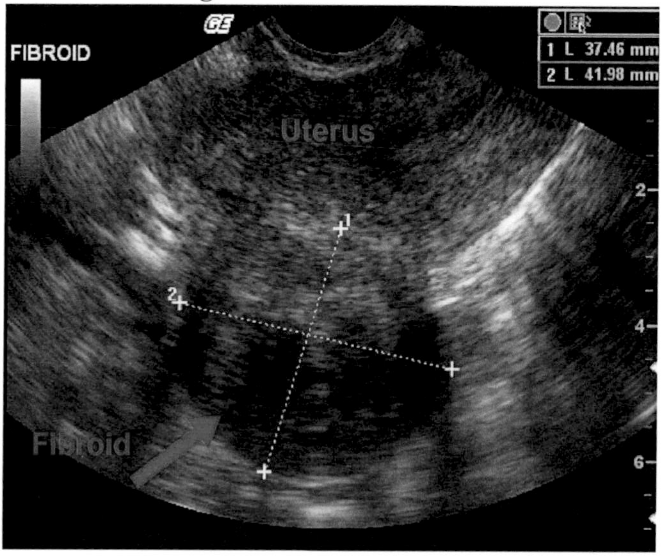

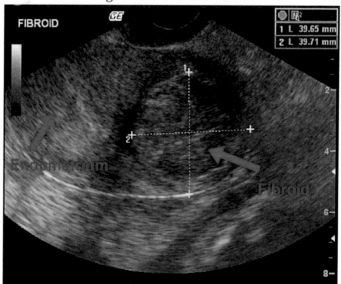

Intramural – Fibroid in the uterine muscle

Figure 4.17 Intramural fibroid

Figure 4.18 Intramural fibroid

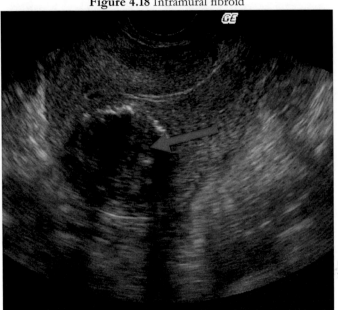

Submucosal – Fibroid in the uterine cavity or lining

Figure 4.19 Submucosal fibroid

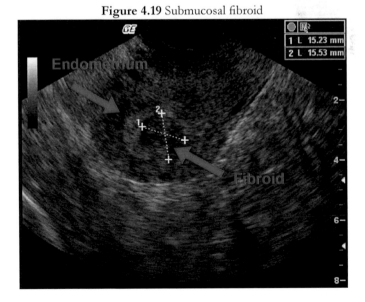

Figure 4.20 Submucosal fibroid

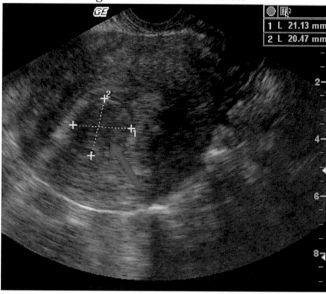

Endometrial polyps

Endometrial polyps are also frequently found in reproductive medicine. A polyp is an overgrowth of tissue located in the lining of the uterus. Many people describe them like a "skin tag" in the uterine cavity. They occur alone or in groups and most are non-cancerous (benign). The problem with polyps is that they may interfere with embryo implantation and may also be related to miscarriages.

When the embryo travels down into the uterus, it may try to implant on the endometrial polyp. Blood flow is compromised on the polyp so the embryo may not implant at all or if it does implant, the lack of blood flow may result in a miscarriage. The good news is that endometrial polyps can be easily removed with a minor outpatient surgical procedure, similar to an egg retrieval or D&C procedure.

Figure 4.21 Endometrial polyp

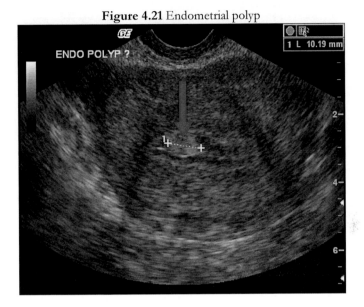

Figure 4.22 Endometrial polyp

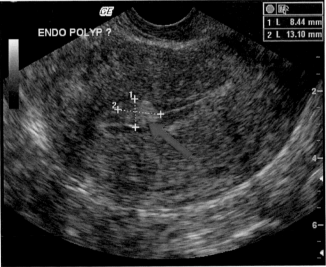

In this image, the endometrium is thick and a possible polyp was noted.

Figure 4.23

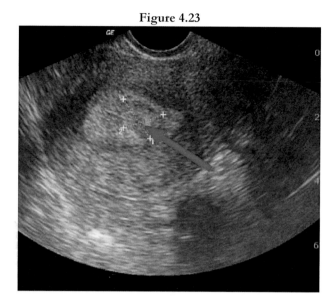

By infusing saline (water) into the uterus, the polyp now becomes more distinct. This is the saline sonohysterogram procedure.

Figure 4.24

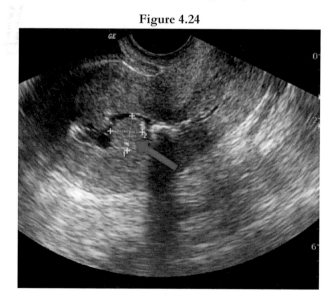

Figure 4.25 Multiple polyps were identified

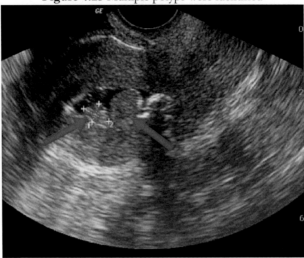

Uterine malformations

Malformations of the uterus can also be identified on ultrasound. Malformations may include uterine didelphys (double uterus), bicornuate uterus (commonly referred to as a "heart-shaped" uterus), or uterine septum (a division in the cavity). These malformations are formed during your own fetal development in utero. Uterine malformations increase the risk of infertility, miscarriage, preterm labor, and fetal growth restriction, depending on the severity of the abnormality. Some uterine malformations may require surgical intervention.

On ultrasound, two separate endometrial cavities are observed. A 3D ultrasound or hysteroscopy is more precise with diagnosing the abnormality.

Ultrasound image of a bicornuate uterus. Can you see the two separate cavities?

Figure 4.26

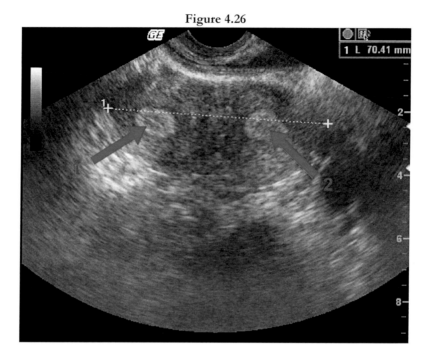

Hydrosalpinx

A hydrosalpinx is the term used to describe a fallopian tube dilated with fluid. The tube may look sausage-like on ultrasound. Fallopian tubes are not routinely seen on ultrasound unless they are fluid filled. The fluid in a hydrosalpinx is detrimental and often described as toxic to a developing embryo. If a hydrosalpinx is identified on ultrasound or on a HSG, it is recommended to either remove or clip the fallopian tube in order to prevent that fluid from leaking down into the uterus.

Ultrasound image of a hydrosalpinx

Figure 4.27 Sausage shape structure

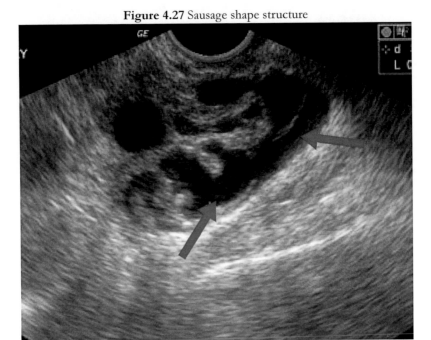

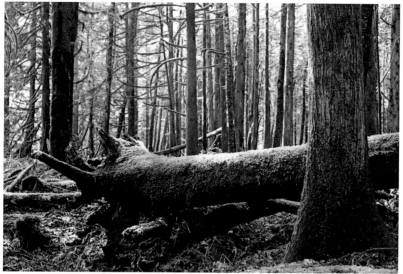

Don't let fallen trees get you off your path.

Rest stop to regroup

We've discussed a variety of cysts, fibroids, and other abnormalities, many of which are frequent occurrences in reproductive medicine. When it occurs to you, however, it feels anything but common. I encourage you to keep taking one step at a time, realizing this could very well be a sidetrack, not a complete derailment in your journey.

Questions for your provider:

Notes:

[i] http://hike-nh.com/faq/glossary/; June 26, 2015

[ii] ibid

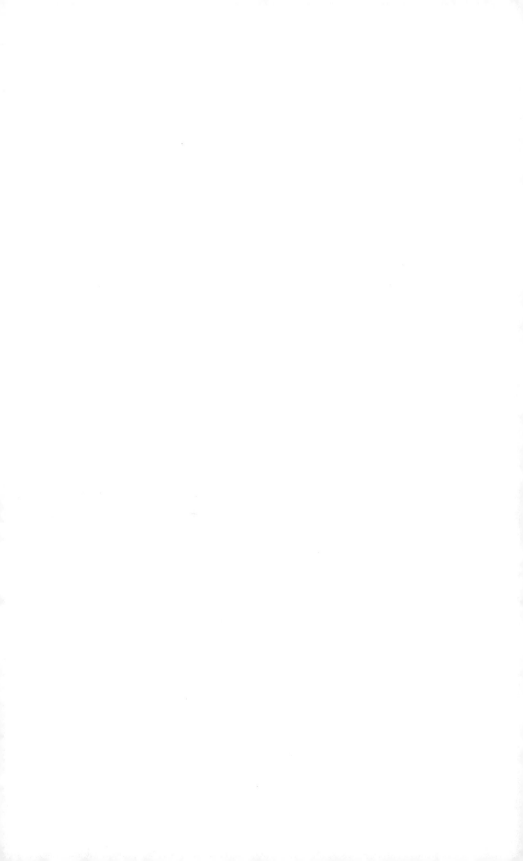

Chapter 5

Treatment Options

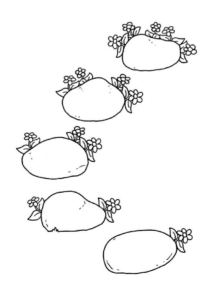

Treatment Options

Ascent: (noun) – A climb or walk to the summit of a mountain or hill.[i]

Traverse: (verb) – To pass along or go across something, in hiking usually a mountain or hillside sloped on one side, or a river.[ii]

Throughout the entire fertility journey, there always seems to be too much information and not enough time. It's no wonder the initial consultation can be difficult for many women treading the path toward fertility. The visit to discuss treatment options can be equally overwhelming. Depending on your medical history and diagnosis, different options may range from simple interventions to advanced reproductive technologies. Other factors influencing your treatment plan include age, ovarian reserve, duration of infertility, costs, and success rates.

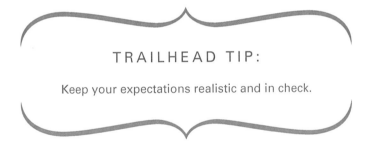

TRAILHEAD TIP:

Keep your expectations realistic and in check.

What's your plan B?

Looking back, the worst part of my fertility journey was the persistent, never-ending emotional roller coaster. I'll never forget the excitement about possible success quickly followed by complete devastation after an unsuccessful cycle. And then we'd start all over again. So often, this walk feels like an uphill battle. Struggling towards fertility can be so physically and emotionally draining; one key towards successful ascent is to have a plan B set up.

It is wonderful when a treatment works the first time, but truthfully, this is often not the case. In order to get through your journey, you need to have realistic and honest discussions with your provider about expectations and success rates. Each treatment option and chance of success with that particular plan should be reviewed and individualized according to your situation. Most centers will advise 2-3 cycles of a particular treatment; if pregnancy is not realized, it is recommended that you change plans or move on to an alternate treatment. The highest chance of success with any treatment is usually within the first 3 cycles before it tends to plateau.

Treatments

Intrauterine insemination (IUI)

An IUI is a relatively simple procedure, somewhat like a Pap smear, and usually takes a few minutes to perform. The sperm sample is washed and placed in a small catheter that is passed through the cervix and into the uterus. The IUI is beneficial by placing the sperm sample directly into the uterus. An IUI aids in mild male factor, cervical factor, unexplained infertility, and donor sperm insemination. The IUI is timed with urine ovulation predictor kits or by ultrasound and measuring a dominant mature follicle (egg). Human Chorionic Gonadotropin (hCG) may also be used to trigger ovulation and time the IUI.

An IUI semen collection is not a semen analysis, and abstinence is usually not recommended prior to the specimen collection.

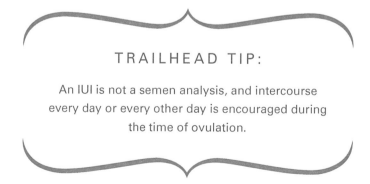

TRAILHEAD TIP:

An IUI is not a semen analysis, and intercourse every day or every other day is encouraged during the time of ovulation.

There is a misperception that frequent ejaculations decrease sperm counts; this is not true, and in fact, intercourse is encouraged — preferably daily or every other day as ovulation approaches.

The highest chance of pregnancy is *before* ovulation with cumulative sperm ready to fertilize the released egg. Ovulation predictor kits are helpful since they turn positive before ovulation has occurred and explains why daily or every other day intercourse is encouraged during the ovulation window (unless otherwise specified by your physician).

Oral fertility medications

Oral fertility medications are often used as a first line of treatment for women with irregular menstrual cycles, unexplained infertility, or mild male factor. The risk of twins is 7-8% higher than normal if more than one follicle is growing. In general, oral fertility medications are well tolerated; however, some women describe their side effects to be worse than injectable medications, citing hot flashes and irritability as the top two culprits.

TRAILHEAD TIP:

The goal of oral fertility medications is to get 1 or 2 mature follicles (eggs) to ovulate.

Figure 5.1 One dominant follicle

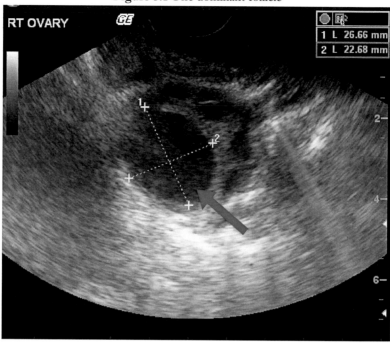

Injectable fertility medications (gonadotropins)

This type of treatment requires closer monitoring with frequent office visits and may include an ultrasound and an estrogen blood test. The pregnancy success rate is a little higher than oral fertility medications; however, there is a much higher risk of a multiple pregnancy.

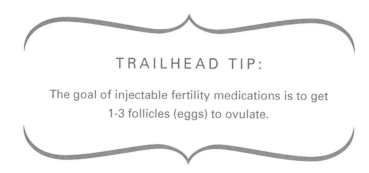

TRAILHEAD TIP:

The goal of injectable fertility medications is to get 1-3 follicles (eggs) to ovulate.

Figure 5.2 Two dominant follicles

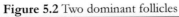

Figure 5.3 Three dominant follicles

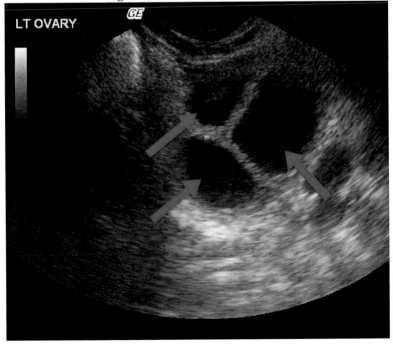

Combination treatment

Another approach is to use a combination of oral agents, starting on day 2 or 3 of the menstrual cycle, and then do low dose injectable medications for 4-5 days. The goal with this type of protocol is to get 2-3 mature follicles (eggs) to ovulate. This method can be useful in older women or when there is male factor infertility.

In vitro fertilization (IVF)

This treatment is very effective for cases such as fallopian tube blockage or moderate to severe male factor. It is also used for unexplained infertility, advanced maternal age, endometriosis, and when other treatments have failed. It is important to understand that success rates are largely determined by age of the woman.

IVF is a process where multiple follicles are stimulated with injectable medications for approximately 8-14 days with the average being 10 days. These days went by quickly for me and I experienced minimal side effects from the medications. The most common symptoms I hear are feeling bloated and tired from the increasing estrogen level. The stimulation medications are given subcutaneously (sub-q) with a tiny needle into your abdomen. The actual egg retrieval is done with an ultrasound, just like the ultrasound used to measure your growing follicles. The only difference is that the ultrasound for the retrieval has a long needle attached used to extract the eggs. This is a minor surgical procedure which takes approximately 20 minutes to perform; however, plan to be at the surgery center for 1-2 hours because of the time allotment needed for anesthesia. Complications are extremely rare; your provider will discuss these and any questions you may have prior to the procedure. The laboratory will look for mature eggs which can either be cryopreserved (frozen) or fertilized. Once fertilization occurs, the embryos will grow in the laboratory until they are ready to be transferred back into the uterus with the hope of implantation. The embryos may also be cryopreserved or biopsied to screen for genetic abnormalities and then transferred back into the uterus in a subsequent cycle.

When infertility becomes personal

Through the years, I've had many patients tell me IVF was their last option or they couldn't imagine doing IVF. When I got married, I never thought I would have to go through advanced reproductive technologies such as these. Conception should occur naturally, right? But what if it doesn't?

My husband and I were in our twenties when we found out we were infertile. It seemed unbelievable to me; yet I determined to learn and understand the science behind infertility. I went back to school to become a Women's Health Care Nurse Practitioner, and I did all of my research on reproductive medicine. I confidently dismissed statements from the doctor such as, "there is nothing we can do."

Technology advanced and seven years later we were told "maybe" instead of "no." We underwent IVF, but my cycle was awful; we almost can-celed the cycle because of my low response. I will never forget the phone call informing us five eggs fertilized, but only four embryos were growing. It is so hard to explain the emotions we went through until I reached the eventual point of "letting go." To this day I struggle to describe that over-powering experience. I remember my mother's words of wisdom grow-ing up. She would say "this too shall pass." I thought about her words and everything we had gone through. It's hard to believe, but I truly was at peace—whatever the outcome.

Our IVF cycle was successful and to this day I wear a pin on my lab coat that states" Believe in Miracles." I looked back at my journal during this time and found an entry dated February 18th, 2001, the day before my scheduled C-section: "Our lives are about to completely change tomorrow – after eight years of dreaming to be parents, our day is finally here!"

Fertility preservation

Fertility preservation is the process of freezing eggs or sperm. In order for eggs to be frozen, the female will have to take ovarian stimulation medications and undergo an egg retrieval procedure as described above (IVF). After the eggs are retrieved, they are cryopreserved (frozen) and stored for future use. If a woman decides to later use her eggs, she will meet with a fertility specialist to review the best way to prepare her uterus for pregnancy. The eggs are then thawed and injected with sperm; the resulting embryo is transferred into the uterus.

IVF and fertility preservation ultrasound

In a normal appearing ovary at a "resting state," antral follicles are counted to assess potential response to the fertility medications and to help your provider determine your medication dose. In this image, 13 antral follicles were counted on the left ovary.

Figure 5.4 Left ovary antral follicle count 13

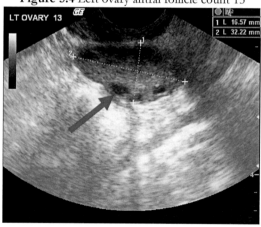

In this normal appearing ovary, 15 antral follicles were counted for a total of 28 follicles. This is an example of a baseline assessment and follicle count can certainly change. The number of follicles could increase or may even decrease if all of the follicles counted do not continue to grow.

Figure 5.5 Right ovary antral follicle count 15

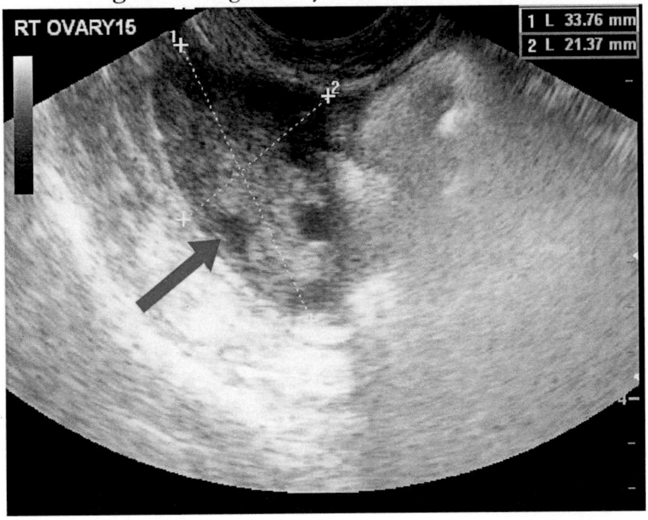

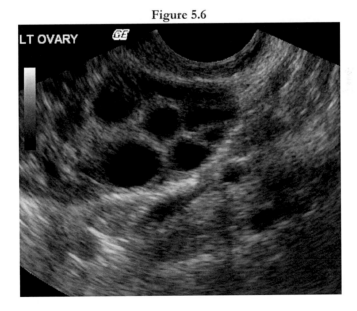

After 5-6 days of injectable medications, you can see how the follicles look larger. The average size of the lead follicles at this time are between 8-10 millimeters.

Figure 5.6

Right ovary, after 5-6 days of injectable medications.

Figure 5.7

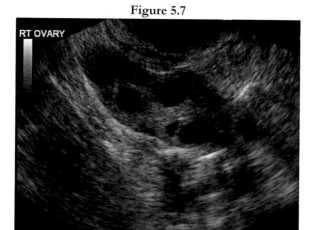

Right ovary – after 9 to 11 days of ovarian stimulation. The lead follicles now measure, on average, 12-18 millimeters.

Figure 5.8

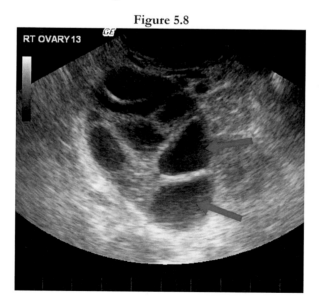

Left ovary – all 28 follicles have grown. The most common side effect at this stage is feeling tired because of the elevated estrogen level and feeling heavy or bloated from the size of the ovaries and fluid retention.

Figure 5.9

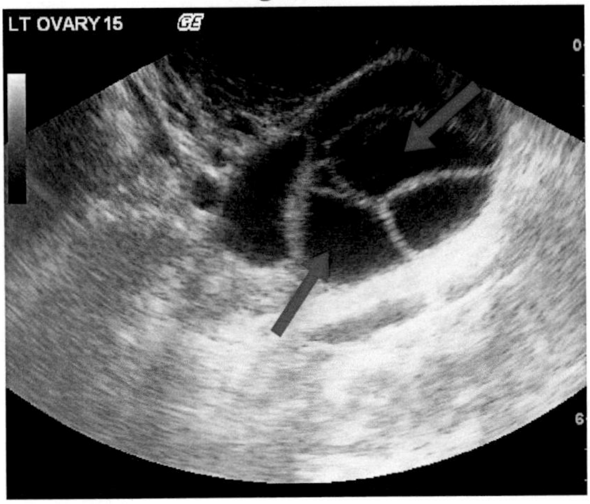

Third party reproduction

Third party cycles may include donor egg, donor sperm, donor embryos, surrogate, or gestational carrier. There are so many wonderful resources within your fertility practice and on various websites regarding third party reproduction that I encourage you to explore. I have seen so many beautiful babies born and such happy families because of this amazing treatment option.

With third party cycles, such as donor egg, donor embryo, or gestational carrier, a main focus is to prepare the uterus for implantation. This can be achieved with either a natural cycle (if normal ovulatory cycles) or with estrogen and progesterone hormone supplementation. Your provider will check your endometrial thickness with an ultrasound. An endometrial thickness of 8 millimeters or more is ideal; however, numerous pregnancies have occurred with an endometrial thickness between 6-8 millimeters.

This next image shows the ultrasound image of a normal endometrial thickness.

Figure 5.10

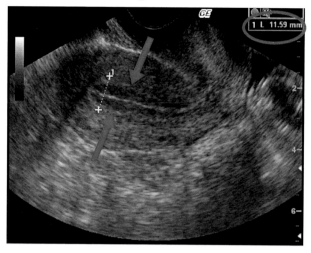

Adoption

Many patients consider adoption but have no idea how to begin. A few good places to start are an adoption exchange resource, a website in your local state, or your state Department of Health and Human Services. These should provide information regarding state requirements as well as a list of adoption agencies. You may decide to work with an agency who will act as your advocate, or you may decide to go through an independent adoption.

My husband and I adopted a little girl, and it has been the most remarkable and rewarding experience, more than we could have ever imagined. We learned so much through that process, I could write an entire book just on adoption. If you are considering this option, my advice is, "Follow your heart." It's not easy though, and we had many tears along the way, but for us, we couldn't envision doing anything else.

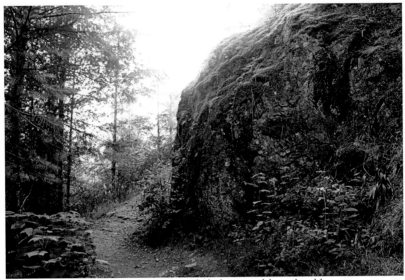

Even though you may feel obstructed by a boulder,
there ARE alternative paths to take.

Rest stop to regroup

It may not seem like it yet, but you've already made significant progress on your fertility walk. It's all perspective, though, isn't it? Right now, maybe all you see are trees (roadblocks), cliffs (dangers), or rocky cliffs (heartache). When you feel overwhelmed about the journey still ahead, be sure to look behind you and appreciate how far you've already come. Here's my encouragement: Don't give up. Take a deep breath. Reorient yourself and take another step.

What treatment options are you already considering?

Which (if any) treatment options seem impossible or not an option for you?

What is your plan B?

Questions for your provider:

Notes:

http://www.oxforddictionaries.com/us/definition/american_english/ascent; June 26, 2015

http://hike-nh.com/faq/glossary/; June 26, 2015

Chapter 6

When Your Pregnancy Test is Positive

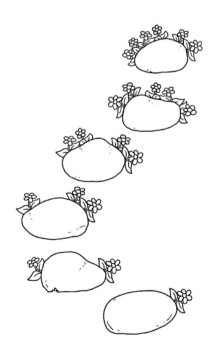

When Your Pregnancy Test is Positive

Bagging the Peak: (verb) – Reaching the summit of a mountain.[i]

Footprint: (noun) – Besides the obvious, "mark your boot leaves," a footprint is the physical space and shape a particular item takes up.[ii]

You're standing at the top, slightly breathless, taking in the scenic beauty around you. The uphill journey has been a difficult one, with setbacks and wrong turns. With the help of your provider, partner (if applicable), friends, and family, you've conquered the mountains of infertility. In many ways, you've conquered other mountains as well: discouragement, fear, anger, fatigue, confusion. Now that you have achieved the goal (pregnancy!), it's good (really!) to set some new ones.

I created this section to help you through questions regarding your pregnancy test and what to do (or not do) through your first 10 weeks of pregnancy. After going through infertility myself, the reality that it actually worked can be a lot to process, and many more questions may suddenly emerge. Consider this a general overview to help guide you on your next adventure.

- What does the serum (blood) hCG level mean?
- Pregnancy dating, early symptoms, and OB referral
- Early OB ultrasound and images
- Diet, medications
- Activity, exercise, intercourse, and travel
- Vaginal bleeding or cramping and when to call

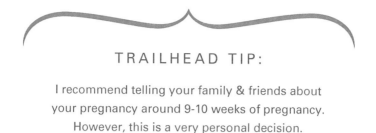

TRAILHEAD TIP:

I recommend telling your family & friends about
your pregnancy around 9-10 weeks of pregnancy.
However, this is a very personal decision.

What does the serum (blood) hCG level mean?

HCG is the abbreviation for "Human Chorionic Gonadotropin," the hormone produced by the placenta as soon as implantation has occurred, typically 8 to 10 days after conception.

The measurement of hCG in a blood test can help assess the viability of a pregnancy. HCG levels rise until about 10-12 weeks of pregnancy, at which point the level will stabilize or drop. In early pregnancy, the hCG doubles (or has an approximate 53-66% rise) every 2-3 days. In a nonviable or **ectopic pregnancy** (a pregnancy outside the uterus), the hCG may have normal levels initially but may increase at a slower rate.

A **biochemical pregnancy**, by definition, is when there is evidence of conception based only on biochemical (hCG) level in the bloodstream or in urine before an ultrasound shows evidence of a pregnancy in the uterus. In a biochemical pregnancy, early embryo development begins but then stops growing, and the hCG level begins to drop. It is estimated that up to 25% of pregnancies in the normal population may be biochemical. A woman may have a late or irregular menstrual cycle and may experience a biochemical pregnancy without ever even knowing it.

Standard pregnancy guidelines for first hCG levels

- *hCG < 5 mIU/ml* is considered negative. Note: some laboratories or providers consider hCG < 10 mIU/ml as negative.

- *hCG 10 - 50 mIU/ml* is a positive result, but this is considered to be on the low side. When the hCG level is low, it may indicate that the pregnancy may not be growing as expected.

- *hCG > 50 mIU/ml* is a good first hCG level.

It is important to repeat the hCG level in 2-3 days as instructed by your provider in order to determine if the pregnancy is a viable pregnancy, a biochemical pregnancy, or an ectopic pregnancy. If the hCG level does not double or rise at least 53%, there may be concern about the outcome of the pregnancy. In general, the hCG blood test only needs to be repeated 1-2 times depending on the results.

Pregnancy dating

A pregnancy is referred to in weeks, starting from the first day of your last menstrual period (LMP). Since ovulation generally occurs about 2 weeks after your period starts, it means that a woman who is 6 weeks pregnant is carrying a 4 week old embryo. Therefore, at the time of your pregnancy test with more precise dates such as in IVF or IUI, you are already considered to be 4 weeks pregnant. This can be quite confusing for infertility patients who know exact dates of conception.

Early pregnancy symptoms

Early pregnancy symptoms are highly variable and can be different from one pregnancy to the next. Some symptoms include slight spotting or mild cramping (like menstrual cramps), heavy or sore breasts, feeling tired, nausea, heightened sense of smell, frequent urination, constipation, mood swings, dizziness, and food aversions or cravings. Some women may have no symptoms at all, which is perfectly okay. Additionally, symptoms may come and go during the first trimester. Many patients are convinced that the decrease in pregnancy symptoms indicates a miscarriage; however, this is not always the case. Typically, I will perform an ultrasound for reassurance and find a completely normal intrauterine pregnancy. I would much rather perform an ultrasound than put my patients through needless worrying.

Obstetrics provider (OB) referral

It is often recommended that you contact your OB provider after confirmation of normally rising hCG blood levels. Most fertility centers will perform your first OB ultrasound between 6-8 weeks of pregnancy. You may also be advised at this time to schedule your first appointment with your OB around 8-12 weeks of pregnancy.

Early pregnancy on ultrasound

The following images are examples of early pregnancy on transvaginal ultrasound.

5 weeks of pregnancy

- The yolk sac is a small sac, attached to the embryo, that can be seen on ultrasound in early pregnancy

- The yolk sac provides early nourishment and functions as the circulatory system before internal circulation begins

- No, this is not the baby's head (yes, I get asked this question a lot)

Figure 6.1 Five weeks

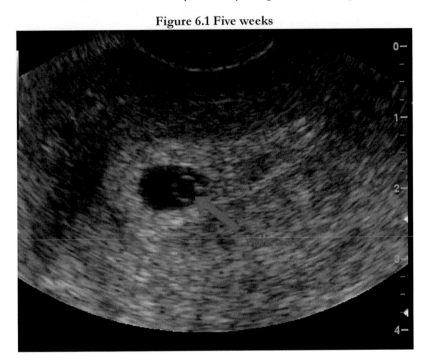

6 weeks of pregnancy

- The embryo is the size of a small bean or a grain of rice

- You may or may not see a heartbeat at 6 weeks

- The heart beat first starts slow, between 80-90 beats per minute (bpm), then there is a rapid rise in early pregnancy during the development of cardiac neuroreceptors, often between 170-175 bpm. It will then decrease at 10-12 weeks of pregnancy to the normal 120-160 bpm.

Figure 6.2 Six weeks

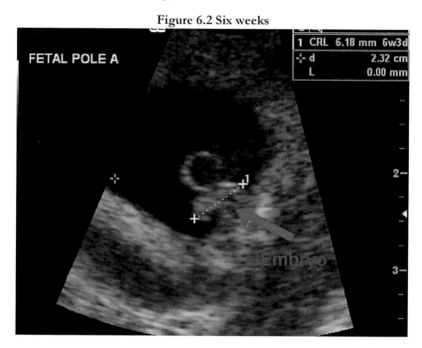

7 weeks of pregnancy

- The fetal heartbeat should be clearly seen at 7 weeks

- The embryo measures about ½ inch long

- The embryo has distinct, slightly webbed fingers and toes

- Protruding buds which will become the arms and legs can begin to be seen on ultrasound

- The embryo has an oversized head in proportion to its body

Figure 6.3 Seven weeks

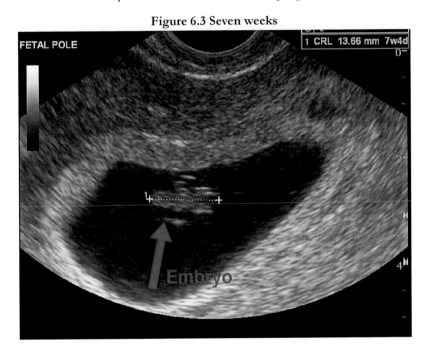

8 weeks of pregnancy

- This week marks the end of the embryonic phase of development and now the embryo is called a fetus

- The fetus is approximately 1 inch long

- All major organs and body systems have begun to develop

- This is my favorite stage to perform an ultrasound; the fetus looks like, and is about the size of, an actual gummy bear with arm and leg buds

Figure 6.4 Eight weeks

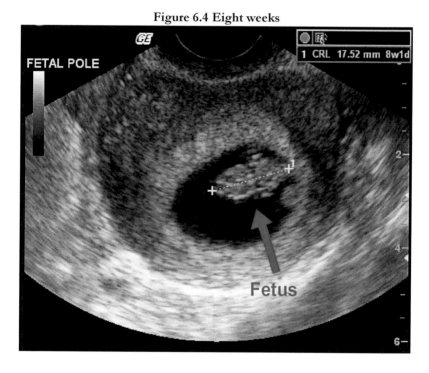

9 weeks of pregnancy

- The placenta, the connection between the mother's blood supply and the fetus, is becoming fully developed

- The development of the skeleton has begun, and the internal reproductive organs have developed

Figure 6.5 Nine weeks

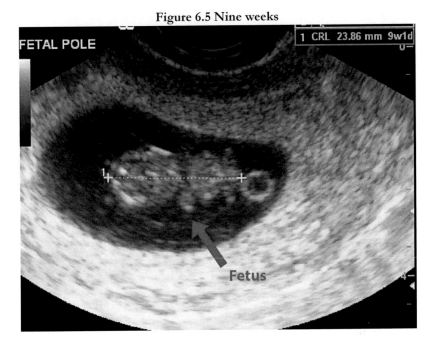

10 weeks of pregnancy

- Fingers and toes continue to grow and soft nails begin to form
- Fetal movement can be easily observed on ultrasound; wiggling all around even though you cannot feel this yet

Figure 6.6 Ten weeks

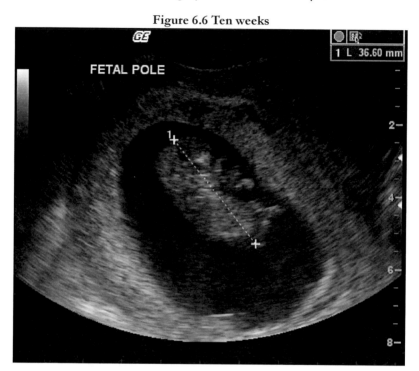

Diet

It is important to eat a well-balanced diet with fresh fruits and vegetables, whole grains, lean proteins, and healthy fats. It is also recommended to avoid or limit caffeine intake to around 200 milligrams per day (1 cup of coffee or tea) and to avoid all forms of alcohol.

Listeria monocytogenes: Listeria is a bacteria that can be found in raw foods and is killed by pasteurization and cooking. Pregnant women should not consume deli-meats (unless reheated), unpasteurized (raw) cheeses, and raw eggs. Avoid uncooked hot dogs or luncheon meats.

Vitamins and supplements: At least 4 servings daily of dairy products are recommended to provide calcium, protein, and vitamin D. The recommended intake of calcium is 1,000 milligrams per day and adequate Vitamin D intake is 600 international units/day, unless a deficiency has been identified. *Do not take more than the recommended daily dietary allowance of any vitamins and minerals.*

Prenatal vitamin and folic acid: It is essential to take a prenatal vitamin with at least 800 micrograms of folic acid daily. Folic acid, also known as folate, may help reduce the risk of neural tube defects that occur when the coverings of the spinal cord do not close completely during prenatal development. Although folic acid is found in many foods, it is often difficult to get the recommended amount from diet alone.

Fish: Fish is an excellent source of protein and healthy fats, but pregnant women should avoid raw fish and high-mercury containing fish which can be neurotoxic to the fetus. Fish with low mercury levels include shrimp, salmon, Pollock, catfish, and tuna but should be limited to 2 servings per week. High mercury fish to be avoided include swordfish, shark, tile fish, and king mackerel. Do not eat raw meat or fish because of the increased risk of parasites.

Lifestyle changes

Smoking: Pregnant women should not smoke and should avoid all second-hand smoke.

Toxoplasmosis: If you own or care for an outdoor cat, do not change the litter box. Cats may carry toxoplasmosis, which is a parasite. If you must change the cat litter, wear gloves. You can also check your titers to see if you have antibodies against toxoplasmosis.

Medications:

- Please continue taking your prenatal vitamin every day
- If you were prescribed estrogen and/or progesterone, you may be instructed to continue these until 10-12 weeks of pregnancy depending on your type of treatment. Your provider will inform you when you can stop the hormone support. Also, your insurance may cover your hormone support after a positive pregnancy test so be sure to check with your pharmacy when ordering refills

While some medications are considered safe to take during pregnancy, the effects of other medications on a fetus are unknown. Therefore, it is very important to pay special attention to medications you take while you are pregnant, especially during the first trimester, a crucial time of development for your baby.

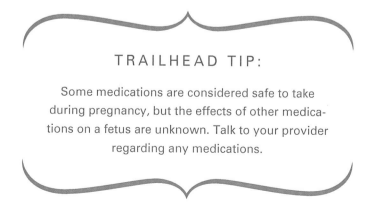

TRAILHEAD TIP:

Some medications are considered safe to take during pregnancy, but the effects of other medications on a fetus are unknown. Talk to your provider regarding any medications.

If you were taking prescription medications before you became pregnant, please discuss them with your health care provider about their safety. Your provider who prescribed the medication will review the medical benefit for you against the risk to your baby. The risk of not taking some medications may be more serious than taking them during pregnancy.

If possible, it is best to avoid all medications and herbal supplements during the first trimester. Please continue your prenatal vitamins and any medications your physician has asked you to take during pregnancy.

Activity, exercise, intercourse, and travel

Feeling tired in early pregnancy is very normal and exercise can boost your energy level. Good options for exercise include walking, low-impact aerobics, swimming, stationary cycling, yoga, Pilates, or toning classes. For most women, the heart rate during exercise should not exceed 140-150 beats per minute (bpm). Training for a marathon or other competitive events or heavy lifting is generally not recommended.

You should avoid hot yoga, intervals, or sprints where your pulse would rise above 150 bpm, or activities where there is a risk of falling, injury, or trauma. You should also avoid exercise if you experience vaginal bleeding when pregnant. Do not go horseback riding, scuba diving, or engage in high-risk sports. Do not go in hot tubs, hot baths, or saunas because they increase core body temperature.

Hair color: No association between hair dye and fetal malformations has been found, but many providers recommend waiting to use these products until after the first trimester.

Intercourse: Having normal sexual intercourse during pregnancy is safe, but I can appreciate the hesitation that something could go wrong. Some women may have a little bleeding after intercourse because the cervix is sensitive, but this does not cause a miscarriage. If you do experience any vaginal bleeding, it is often recommended to abstain from intercourse until you have been seen by your provider to prevent any further irritation.

Dental work: Preventive dental cleanings and annual exams during pregnancy are safe and recommended because the rise in hormone levels during pregnancy can cause the gums to swell, bleed, and trap food. Preventive dental work while pregnant helps to avoid oral infections, such as gum disease, which have been linked to preterm birth. It is important to let your dentist know you are pregnant and discuss any additional dental work if necessary.

Travel: In general, travel during pregnancy is safe unless otherwise advised by your provider. It is recommended to take frequent walking breaks, stay hydrated, and avoid heavy lifting. The American College recommends no air travel after 33 weeks or around 7 months of pregnancy.

Vaccinations: The Centers for Disease Control and Prevention (CDC) recommends two vaccinations during pregnancy (if you have not already been vaccinated before pregnancy). This includes the Flu vaccine and Tdap. Pregnant women can get the flu shot, which is made with killed viruses. Do not, however, get the Nasal spray flu vaccine, which contains live viruses. Tdap (tetanus, diphtheria and pertussis) is also recommended if you have not already had the vaccine prior to pregnancy. It can be given after 20 weeks of pregnancy.

Vaginal bleeding and cramping

Any vaginal bleeding during early pregnancy can be alarming and may cause a great deal of anxiety. I panicked and cried all night the first time I bled during my early pregnancy. My husband and I were out at a movie theater when I felt this warm gush of fluid. I went to the restroom and found that I was soaked in blood. I walked back into the theater and told my husband, "We are leaving now." We never did see the end of that movie, and I put myself on bed rest through the rest of that weekend.

It is so terrifying to experience any vaginal bleeding after going through fertility treatment, but the reassuring news is that vaginal bleeding and cramping in the first trimester of pregnancy is relatively common.

In fact, it occurs in approximately 20-30% of all pregnancies. The amount of bleeding may vary from light spotting to heavy bleeding with clots. The bleeding may be caused by different factors, which are described below.

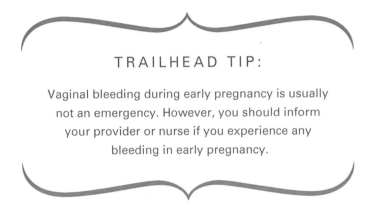

TRAILHEAD TIP:

Vaginal bleeding during early pregnancy is usually not an emergency. However, you should inform your provider or nurse if you experience any bleeding in early pregnancy.

NOTE: When the embryo has created its own red blood cells, vaginal bleeding can lead to the mixing of the mother's and fetal blood. If your blood type is RH negative, an injection of Rhogam will be needed within 3 days of any bleeding. Please contact your provider's office.

Miscarriage: Any bleeding in early pregnancy is termed medically as a "threatened miscarriage." The bleeding may be a sign of a miscarriage, but it does NOT mean that a miscarriage will for sure happen.[iii]

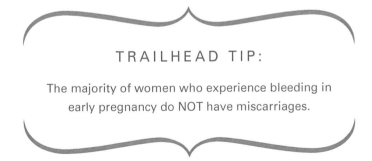

TRAILHEAD TIP:

The majority of women who experience bleeding in early pregnancy do NOT have miscarriages.

Other symptoms of a miscarriage may include cramping, which is stronger than menstrual cramps and passing tissue or blood clots. Going through a miscarriage is an extremely emotional experience but know that most miscarriages cannot be prevented, nor were related to anything you could have possibly done. In most cases, a miscarriage results from an embryo that was chromosomally abnormal and not compatible with life. This is a difficult time but keep in mind that this does NOT mean that you cannot have a future healthy pregnancy.

Ectopic pregnancy: This is a pregnancy that implants outside the uterus. The most common site for an ectopic pregnancy is in the fallopian tube. As the embryo grows, it can rupture the tube and cause life-threatening bleeding. Ectopic pregnancies are much less common than a miscarriage. Signs of an ectopic pregnancy may include cramping that is stronger than menstrual cramps, abdominal pain, abnormal hCG levels, vaginal bleeding, shoulder pain, and lightheadedness. If you experience any of these symptoms, you should contact your provider immediately.

Subchorionic hematoma: This is the term used to describe pooling of blood or "blood clot" between the uterine wall and the developing placenta. Although this may cause significant concern, most subchorionic hematomas will resolve spontaneously. If you have been diagnosed with this, your provider may recommend limited activity, pelvic rest, and no intercourse. There is nothing you did to cause the hematoma and unfortunately, there are no medical interventions or medications to make it go away. The recommendation is usually to just watch and wait with follow-up ultrasounds, which, understandably, is emotionally very difficult.

Intercourse: Some women may have a little bleeding after intercourse because the cervix is sensitive, but this does not cause a miscarriage. If you do experience any vaginal bleeding, it is often recommended to abstain from intercourse to prevent any further irritation.

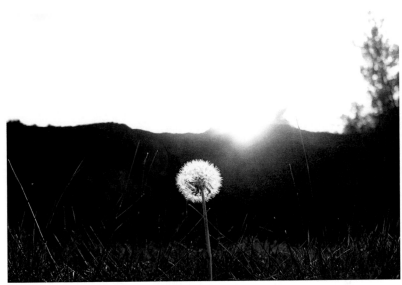

You just want to hold your breath.

Rest stop to regroup

Just because you're pregnant, doesn't mean you need to have everything figured out; descending from the mountaintop will present its own set of challenges, concerns—and celebrations! The impact (or footprint) this new tiny person will make on your life is monumental. Stay diligent and focused, remembering that as mothers we can tend to overthink (and over-worry!) things. Parenthood is another walk/trudge/hike/crawl, one that can take many different paths. Remember to enjoy your child as the unique individual he or she will become.

Questions for your provider:

Notes:

---

[i] http://hike-nh.com/faq/glossary/; June 26, 2015.

[ii] Ibid.

[iii] http://americanpregnancy.org/pregnancy-complications/miscarriage

Chapter 7

Taking One Day at a Time

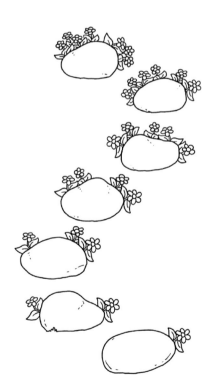

Taking One Day at a Time

FPA: (noun) - Forest Protection Area. Formerly called RUAs. An area where camping, camp fires, and travel are restricted to allow the area to recover from overuse.[i]

Fiver: (noun) – A 5 minute break.[ii]

Keeping yourself sane through this time in your life

Whether you are freezing your eggs for fertility preservation or are actively trying to get pregnant, this particular stage in your life can be extremely taxing on your relationships, home life, finances, etc. Perhaps you need an extra rest, or a metaphorical "fiver" on this journey. You alone know your body, your heart, and your stress. I encourage you to be aware of the toll this fertility walk can and will take on your life.

I can't emphasize enough the importance of setting aside time with your partner (if applicable), time away from the trail; allow yourselves time to recover from "overuse." Be sure to set boundaries for yourselves to avoid burnout.

Bear in mind this is a journey, and although it may feel like it has taken over your life, I promise it will not last forever. As I mentioned earlier, my mother reminded me during difficult times, "This too shall pass." I remember feeling the impossibility of that statement at the moment, but she was right.

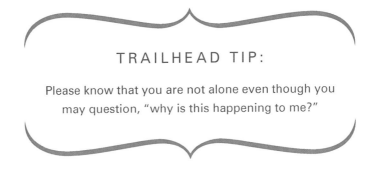

TRAILHEAD TIP:

Please know that you are not alone even though you may question, "why is this happening to me?"

Several studies show the tension of fertility treatment can be comparable to the stress of serious or life-threatening illness, and the primary reason for stopping treatment is patient distress, not doctor recommendation, or financial constraints.

Developing strategies for coping with the ups and downs may enable you to make decisions to help reach your ultimate goal of parenting. It is completely normal to feel frustrated at times and question why this is happening to you. It is also natural to have significant sadness since this may not be what you ever imagined for your life. This sorrow is without doubt even more profound when a cycle fails or when it results in a miscarriage.

While in the midst of infertility treatments, it is easy to become preoccupied with every detail about your menstrual cycle and obsessed with every single symptom you may experience. Sexual intimacy may also take a toll, and intercourse may feel rigid with loss of spontaneity. It is not uncommon to go through the gamut of emotions—sadness, irritability, frustration—sometimes all in the same day! Besides the stress, the hormones alone can drive you crazy.

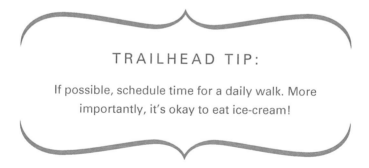

TRAILHEAD TIP:

If possible, schedule time for a daily walk. More importantly, it's okay to eat ice-cream!

To my fellow traveler on this weary, rugged, sometimes lonely path,
My HOPE for you is . . .
To trust that this too shall pass
To not let infertility take over your life
To stay strong through the good and the bad
To believe you CAN achieve your dreams even though the paths may change along the way
Let's continue our walk together . . .

Writing can be a good way to explore your private thoughts and feelings and can help reduce stress. I encourage you use the questions below as a guide to unlock your personal concerns associated with fertility treatment. You may be as elaborate as you wish or simply jot down one-word thoughts.

To help get you started, I thought I would share with you a few entries from my own journal. Even though it has been many years, I believe these same thoughts and feelings still resonate:

- *In my heart, I am truly happy for my younger sister who is pregnant. I love her dearly, but in my mind, I am jealous and so deeply saddened. Now both my brother and his wife, my sister and her husband are having babies. Tim and I, who were the first married in our family, still have no kids. I cannot stop my tears, sadness, and feeling so alone.*

- *I feel so isolated. My family stopped asking about babies after 5 years into our marriage. It's been a mixed blessing to live out of state at this time, since it's just too hard to be at family gatherings and baby showers. I can tell everyone that I'm busy with work and school and maybe they won't ask. What hurts even more is when my own family member didn't tell us that they were pregnant until 5 months into their pregnancy. I can understand that it's hard for all of us, but the feeling of being deliberately left out is so painful.*

- *It feels like everyone around me is pregnant. Even though I know this is not true, it's hard to convince by brain of anything else. I keep asking, "Why?" "Why is this happening?" Every time my period starts, I feel like such a failure and I'm so depressed.*

- *I wish I could talk to Tim more about my feelings, but it always ends up in a fight.*

Do any of these thoughts and feelings sound familiar? If so, please know that you are not alone, and these ways of thinking are so common with those struggling with reproductive issues.

When it becomes too much

Often we try to do too much and think we are just fine. But, the following signs (below) may signal that we need a walking partner such as a fertility counselor or social worker to keep us on the right path. These may include:

- Decreased optimism about getting pregnant
- Increased anxiety, depression, or sadness that is taking over your life
- Increased social isolation and avoiding friends and family

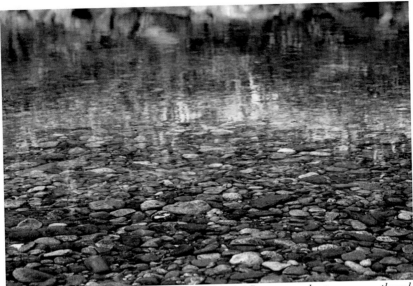

I have stared into these waters and pondered. Nature speaks to me even though no words are spoken.

A Final rest stop to regroup

Keeping yourself sane through this time in your life can be a challenge. Nevertheless, you are not alone. Seek out friends, family, and professional support – whatever it takes. Take a little time every day to jot down your thoughts. You will be amazed with how far you've come when you look back on your notes later. I promise, you WILL get through this.

Journaling Questions

What are some of your fears?

What situations make you feel stressed and what are some strategies you can do to help?

The hormonal roller coaster can be so difficult. What can you do to manage these ups & downs?

What is your dream? Are there ways in which this dream is creating more stress for you now?

---

[i] http://hike-nh.com/faq/glossary/; June 26, 2015.

[ii] Ibid.

Resources

American Society for Reproductive Medicine (ASRM)

www.asrm.org

Centers for Disease Control and Prevention (CDC)

www.cdc.gov/ART/index.htm

Society for Assisted Reproductive Technology (SART)

www.sart.org

National Institute of Child Health and Human Development (NICHD)

www.nichd.nih.gov

RESOLVE: The National Infertility Association

www.resolve.org

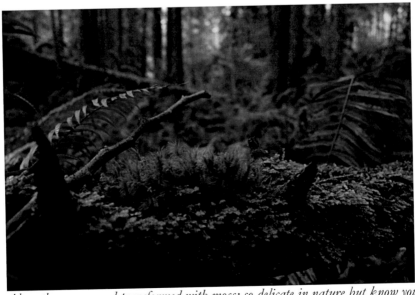

Alone these years and transformed with moss; so delicate in nature but know you don't have to be alone.

References

1. Allison J, Sherwood R, Schust D. Management of first trimester pregnancy loss can be safely moved into the office. Obstet Gynecol. 2011; 4(1): 5–14.

2. Asato K, Mekaru K, Heshiki C, Sugiyama H, Kiniyo T, Masamoto H, Aoki Y. Subchorionic hematoma occurs more frequently in in vitro fertilization pregnancy. European Journ of OBstes Gynecol 2014;181:41-44.

3. Ashton, Jennifer. Benign Lesions of the Ovaries. http://www.emedicine.com/med/topic3305.htm.

4. Bagratee JS, Khullar V, Regan L, et al. A randomized controlled trial comparing medical and expectant management of first trimester miscarriage. Hum Reprod. 2004;19:266–271.

5. Bauman J. Basal **body temperature**: unreliable method of ovulation detection. Fertility & Sterility 1981; December; 36:729-733.

6. Beall, Stephanie. History and challenges surrounding ovarian stimulation in the treatment of infertility. Fertility & Sterility 2012. April;97:795-801.

7. Behre H, Kuhlage J, Gabner C, Sonntag B, Schem C, Schneider H, Nieschlag E. Prediction of ovulation by urinary hormone measurements with the home use ClearPlan® Fertility Monitor: comparison with transvaginal ultrasound scans and serum hormone measurements. Human Reproduction 2000; December; 15:2478-2482.

8. Body Planes, Public Domain image available at: http://training.seer.cancer.gov/module_anatomy/unit1_3_terminology2_planes.html

9. Bourne T, and Bottomley C. When is a pregnancy nonviable and what criteria should be used to define miscarriage? Fertil Steril 2012;98:1091-1096.

10. Chung K, Sammel M, Coutifaris C, Chalian R, Lin K, Castelbaum A, et al. Defining the rise of serum HCG in viable pregnancies achieved through use of IVF. Hum Reprod 2006;21:823-828.

11. Cole L, Ladner D, Byrn F. The normal variability of the menstrual cycle. Fertility & Sterility 2009; February; 91:522-527.

12. Curran D, Ashton, JL. Benign Lesions of the Ovaries. Medscape Reference Web site. http://www.emedicine.com/med/topic3305.htm.

13. Devoto L, Fuentes A, Kohen P, Cespedes P, Palomino A, Pommer R, Munoz A, Strauss J. The human corpus luteum: life cycle and function in natural cycles. Fertility & Sterility 2008; Article in Press.

14. Fehring R, Schneider M, Raviele K. Variability in the phases of the menstrual cycle. Journal of Obstetric, Gynecologic, & Neonatal Nursing 2006; May; 35:376-384

15. Fleisher A, Kepple D, Herbert III C, Hill G. Transvaginal Sonography in Gynecologic Infertility. Chapter 12, 243.

16. Fleischer, AC, Lin EC. Malignant ovarian tumor imaging. Medscape Reference Web site. http://www.emedicine.com/radio/topic511.htm

17. Fleischer, AC. Sonography in Gynecology and Obstetrics: Just the Facts. New York, NY McGraw Hill Higher Education; 2004.

18. Gariepy A, and Stanwood N. Medical management of early pregnancy failure. Contemporary OB GYN 2013; May 26-33.

19. Goldstein, Ruth B. Ultrasonography in Obstetrics and Gynecology. Chapter 7, 83-98.

20. Green, AE. Borderline ovarian cancer borderline tumor overview. Medscape Reference Web site. http://www.emedicine.com/med/topic3233.htm

21. Hansotia M, Desai S, Parihar M. Advanced Infertility Management 2002.

22. Kyser, Kathy. Meta-analysis of subchorionic hemorrhage and adverse pregnancy outcomes. Proc Obste Gynecol 2012;2(4):;Article 4 (9p.).

23. McGovern P. The unreliability of home urine luteinizing hormone test kits has important implications for clinical practice. Fertility & Sterility 2004; November; 82:1300.

24. Miller P, Soules M. The usefulness of a urinary LH kit for ovulation prediction during menstrual cycles of normal women. Obstetrics & Gynecology 1996; 87:13-17.

25. Moghissi, K. Accuracy of basal body temperature for ovulation detection. Fertility & Sterility 1976; 27:1415-1445.

26. Nyberg DA, Hill LM, Böhm-Vélez M, Mendelson EB, eds. Transvaginal Ultrasound. St. Louis, MO: Mosby-Year Book; 1992.

27. Nyberg D and Filly R. Predicting pregnancy failure in 'empty' gestational sacs. Ultrasound in Obstetrics and Gynecology 2003; 21: 9-12.

28. Park S, Goldsmith L, Skurnick J, Wojtczuk A, Weiss, G. Characteristics of the urinary luteinizing hormone surge in young ovulatory women. Fertility & Sterility 2007; September; 88:684-690.

29. Parker, William. Etiology, symptomatology, and diagnosis of uterine myomas. Fertility and Sterility 2007; April; 87 (4): 725-736.

30. Practice Committee of the American Society for Reproductive Medicine. Use of exogenous gonadotropins in anovulatory women: a technical bulletin. Fertility & Sterility 2008. November; 90:S7-S12.

31. Practice Committee of the American Society for Reproductive Medicine. The clinical relevance of Luteal phase deficiency: a committee opinion. Fertility & Sterility 2012. November; 98: 1112-1117.

32. Practice Committee of the American Society for Reproductive Medicine. Current evaluation of amenorrhea. Fertility & Sterility 2008. November; 90:S219-S225.

33. Practice Committee of the American Society for Reproductive Medicine. Medical treatment of ectopic pregnancy: a committee opinion. Fertil Steril 2013;100:638-644.

34. Rotterdam ESHRE/ASRM – sponsored PCOS Consensus Workshop Group. Fertility and Sterility 2004; January; 81 (1): 19-25.

35. Seeber, Beata. What serial hCG can tell you, and cannot tell you, about an early pregnancy. Fertil Steril 2012;98:1074-1077.

36. Silva c, Sammel M, Zhou L, Gracia C, Hummel A, Barnhart K. Human chorionic gonadotropin profile for women with ectopic pregnancy. Obset Gynecol 2006;107:605-610.

37. Spence A, Mason E. Human Anatomy and Physiology 3rd Edition 1987. Chapter 16, 28, and 29.

38. Speroff L, Glass R, Kase N. Clinical Gynecologic Endocrinology and Infertility. Sixth Edition 1999.

39. Steinkampf MP, Guzick DS, Hammond KR. Identification of early pregnancy landmarks by transvaginal sonography: Analysis by logistic regression. Fertility and Sterility, 68(1), 168, 1997.

40. Teng, N, Simons EJ. Adenxal Tumors. Medscape Reference Web site. http://www.emedicine.com/med/topic2830.htm.

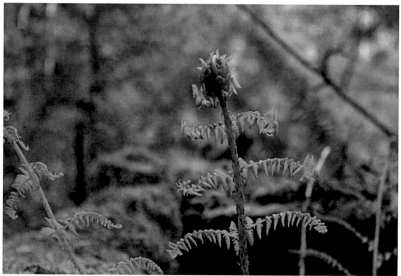

Each time you go into the woods, there is more to discover and learn.

Common
Fertility Abbreviations

AFC –	Antral Follicle Count
AH –	Assisted Hatching
AMH –	Anti-Mullerian Hormone
ART –	Assisted Reproductive Technologies
BBT –	Basal Body Temperature
BCP or OC –	Birth Control Pills/Oral Contraceptive
CCS –	Comprehensive Chromosome Screening
CD –	Cycle Day
CM –	Cervical Mucus
COH –	Controlled Ovarian Hyperstimulation
DE or DEP –	Donor Egg/Donor Egg Program
DOR –	Diminished Ovarian Reserve
E2 –	Estradiol
EMB –	Endometrial Biopsy
ENDO –	Endometriosis
EOC –	Elective Oocyte (Egg) Cryopreservation
eSET –	Elective Single Embryo Transfer
ET –	Embryo Transfer
FD –	Follicular Dynamics
FET –	Frozen Embryo Transfer
FHR –	Fetal Heart Rate
FSH –	Follicle Stimulating Hormone
GnRH –	Gonadotropin Releasing Hormone
hCG –	Human Chorionic Gonadotropin
hMG –	Human Menopausal Gonadotropin
HPT –	Home Pregnancy Test

HRT –	Hormone Replacement Therapy
HSC –	Hysteroscopy
HSG –	Hysterosalpingogram
ICI –	Intra-cervical Insemination
ICSI –	Intracytoplasmic Sperm Injection
IUI –	Intrauterine Insemination
IVF –	In-Vitro Fertilization
LH –	Lutenizing Hormone
LMP –	Last Menstrual Period
LPD –	Luteal Phase Defect
OH/HSC –	Office Hysteroscopy/Hysteroscopy
OHSS –	Ovarian Hyperstimulation Syndrome
OI –	Ovulation Induction
OPK –	Ovulation Predictor Kit
OV –	Ovulation
PCOS –	Polycystic Ovarian Syndrome
PGD –	Preimplantation Genetic Diagnosis
PGS –	Preimplantation Genetic Screening
POF –	Premature Ovarian Failure
P4 –	Progesterone
PIO –	Progesterone in Oil
PRL –	Prolactin
RE –	Reproductive Endocrinologist
SA –	Semen Analysis
SAB –	Spontaneous Abortion (miscarriage)
SC, subQ –	Subcutaneous Injection
SER or ER –	Sonographic Egg Recovery/Egg Retrieval
SIS/SHG –	Saline Sonohysterogram
Supp Check –	Suppression Check Ultrasound
TDI/DI –	TherapeuticDonor Insemination/ Donor Insemination
US –	Ultrasound

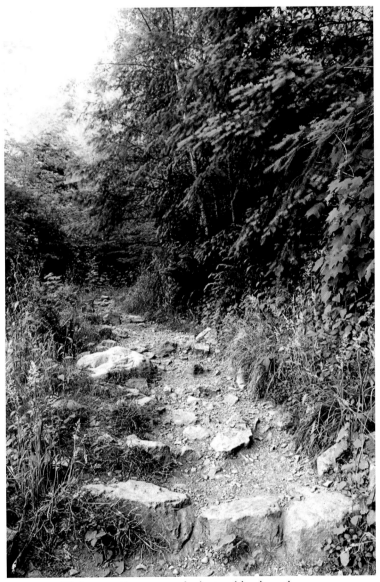

Take your time so you don't stumble along the way.

Nature does not hurry.

www.FertilityWalk.com

My HOPE is that every person struggling with fertility issues will have the opportunity to read this book and better understand their ultrasounds, menstrual cycle, treatment options, and procedures. Proceeds from this book benefit the **Fertility Walk Hope Fund** for those who need fertility treatment but do not have insurance coverage and are financially restricted.

The other purpose of my book is to walk with you along your journey. I would love to hear from you and offer support, encouragement, latest technology updates, etc. For information on the **Fertility Walk Hope Fund** or to follow my blog, please join me at www.FertilityWalk.com.

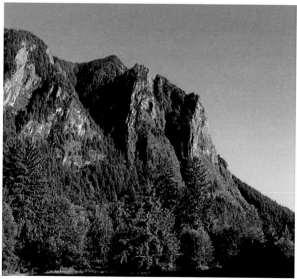

They say the secret in nature is patience.
Embrace stillness and its beauty.